Watchers And Tellers

By

John B. Hill

ISBN: 1-4033-1358-X (e-book)
ISBN: 1-4033-1359-8 (Paperback)

This book is printed on acid free paper.

1stBooks - rev. 06/21/02

For Lainey

FALL

"Yuck!" Jim exclaimed. "It's depressing coming back here after vacation." Returning, in the fall of 1957, to the Medical School on the state operated Wilder University, North Carolina campus, he scowled at the mass of items lying on his desk.

Donna Beardsley, his lab technician, had run his experiments, sorted the lab results and his mail in his absence.

"Dr. Kulp, you've been gone six weeks!" Donna responded. "What did you expect?"

Jim, Janet, his wife, and their four children had combined a cross-country camping trip with Jim's attendance of a pharmacology meeting in San Francisco.

"I'm not critical of you, Donna. It's just the post-vacation letdown. I seem to have one annually. I guess it's a conditioned response to my dislike of going back to school."

She shook her head. "How did you ever manage to get your medical and research degrees?" Seeing that he had begun to rummage through the piles on his desk and probably would ignore or hadn't heard her question, she continued, "This message from the Dean's office came in this morning." She handed him an envelope and left his office.

Jim opened it and was surprised to find not the usual mimeographed announcements, but a personal letter from Dean Mackenzie appointing him to a search committee for the selection of a new head for his own department.

Though Jim knew Professor Mettlar resigned the Pharmacology Chairmanship before he started his cross-country vacation, he had pushed that disheartening fact out of his mind in order to have a decent vacation. He liked and admired Bob Mettlar and dreaded the thought of a replacement.

Dr. Mettlar, head of the Pharmacology Department when Jim came to the University, was a conscientious careful scientist and, in Jim's opinion, an excellent department head and administrator. Honest, intelligent and entirely lacking in artifice, because of extreme shyness, Professor Mettlar was widely considered cold and aloof. He could be warm and outgoing if one made the initial efforts to befriend him, but it was impossible for him to reach out toward others. Jim had made the initial moves and had been rewarded with the friendship of one whose intellect and integrity he respected. For Jim, Professor Robert Mettlar represented all that was good in Science.

Professor Mettlar's pursuit of excellence and his original thinking often brought him into conflict with the dour Dean who had the nasty habit of berating dissenting faculty members in public. A proud man, Professor Mettlar eventually became so unhappy that his resignation as department head was inevitable. His reputation as a researcher in his field was widely respected and he obtained a lifetime investigator grant from the federal government and, thus, could continue research without the daily indignities heaped upon him in his position as department head. His resignation solved Professor Mettlar's problem, but it left the department and the school without a Pharmacology Chairman.

The Dean's letter not only further depressed; but also puzzled him, as he was not aware of any other Search Committee having a member of the department among those choosing a departmental head. Jim, an assistant professor, was a junior member of the Pharmacology Department which taught medical, dental, nursing and pharmacy students about drugs, their uses and abuses.

Jim knocked and entered his former chief's office. Professor Mettlar sat pencil in hand staring at the ceiling. On his ever neat desk lay a yellow pad on which he wrote. Once he put pencil to paper he never changed a thing and woe be to the reviewer or editor who tried to meddle with the syntax in his publications. His conversation, too, tended to be composed of complete grammatical sentences. He was a tall, lean man with piercing blue eyes, blond wavy hair and fine strong features of a Lincoln-like, rugged quality.

"Why Jim, you're back from vacation," he said in a startled manor as he swung his swivel chair round to face him.

"Have you seen this?" Jim asked handing him the Dean's letter.

Professor Mettlar read the letter. "I do not know what Dean Mackenzie has in mind?" Mettlar mused.

"Maybe he wants me to act as liaison between the department and the committee," Jim replied.

"Perhaps, but that would be unusual. Departments have no choice in the matter other than suggesting candidates." He shook his head thoughtfully and stared at the ceiling.

"What will I be doing exactly? I've never been on a selection committee," Jim asked.

Professor Mettlar shrugged. "You'll meet and compose a list of candidates which you'll sift through and select a few to interview. Then, when you make an offer which one accepts, we will have a new department head. Ordinarily it takes six months to a year. I notice in that letter that there are some long-winded members who will be choosing with you. Don't expect an early selection."

"Oh, God," Jim mumbled. "My research goes slowly enough as is. This won't speed it up any."

"True," Professor Mettlar sympathized. "Perhaps you can play a steadying role on the committee and assure a reasonable choice for my successor. If you can, your time will have been well spent. Tony has been holding down the fort as acting head and will be glad to be relieved of that responsibility."

Professor Mettlar was referring to Dr. Anthony Lewis, a full professor and acting head when Professor Mettlar had been hired seven years previously. Jim knew Tony would not be relieved and would prefer being the real and not the acting head, but had little hope for that appointment as his efforts went more into teaching than research which was all-important as far as recognition and advancement were concerned.

If anyone from within the department were to be seriously considered for the position, Jim felt it would be Rodney Barret.

Rodney, an able researcher, was young, ambitious, and hardworking. He had come to Wilder from an excellent department in a Midwestern medical school where he had received a fine training. Jim liked

Rodney, considered him a good friend and felt he would make an excellent successor to Bob Mettlar. If no clearly superior outsider were found, Rodney Barret would be Jim's first choice.

Marie Barret stood on the sidewalk waiting for the light to change. She felt poorly. Cold rain pelted her eyeglasses and added to her misery. Her nausea and headache had been growing steadily since she awoke early that September morning and she was limited in taking headache medicines. As her doctor, Peter Markley, had explained, her kidneys were functioning badly and what would be a normal dose for a well person could prove harmful for her. She dreaded these visits to the hospital which were becoming more and more frequent. Her condition was getting worse. The periods in which she felt really well were fewer and fewer. She was rapidly losing interest in things which had previously been important to her: her home, her family, her warm relationship with Rodney of whom she was intensely proud.

She had married him over her parents objections, feeling that someday they, too, would see what an excellent choice he had been. Older than Rodney by two years, she spared no efforts to help his career as a scientist. She had worked so that he could obtain his doctorate and continued to do so when he chose a post doctorate position in a prestigious and, therefore, low-paying university. When they came to Wilder University, she stopped working and started a family; still she did without many luxuries she'd had while growing up in order to make Rodney's moderate salary serve their needs. Her parents had never forgiven her for marrying out of her faith—she was raised as a Catholic—and did not help her financially although she was an only child. Suddenly she was aware the light had changed. She crossed the street and entered Wilder General Hospital.

The lobby was its usual early morning hodgepodge of humanity. The terrazzo floor was dotted with wet, slippery areas where the rain water tracked in from outside. To help avoid accidents, long black rubber mat pathways crossed the lobby and lethargic mop-wielders from the housekeeping department dabbed here and there to remove the major puddles. Marie, knowing her way, was able to avoid the ever present lines of patients seeking aid in the beginning of a day of shuffling and waiting to see the healer or healers who would allay their fears and solve their problems. She entered the long corridor which traversed the hospital from end to end and sought the Nephrology Clinic where patients with kidney problems are evaluated and treated and where she had her appointment.

The clinic magazine supply was uninspiring but, even had it been current, Marie was unable to concentrate. She was on the verge of tears when the clinic nurse called her name, took her to a small examining room and presented her with a hospital gown. She put it on, sat on the examining table and felt even more miserable. The gown was skimpy and she felt alternately chilled and overly warm. The nurse returned, took her to be weighed and checked her blood pressure. She returned to her perch on the examining table to await Dr. Markley.

Marie had not realized that during her past visits the third-year medical students had been on vacation. Now as she watched the entrance made by a nervous young man in the white twill jacket, she remembered she had been told that medical students would be following her case as they followed all cases in this teaching hospital. Though she was in no mood for any extra discomfort, she recognized the need and approved of a teaching hospital which treated the rich and poor alike.

"I'm Dr. Michaelson, Mrs. Barret. The youngster's appealing smile partially masked his discomfort as he began to take Marie's history. His inexperience, which necessitated frequent referrals to notes to find the proper question to ask, helped Marie to forget, momentarily, her own troubles. They explored her occupational history and Michaelson was surprised to learn she had been a research technician. He wanted to try research himself and through this tenuous bond they began a less strained conversation in which he suddenly realized she was Professor Barret's wife. He had finished his Pharmacology course just last spring and was seeking a senior thesis advisor in that department. During their conversation, he confided to her that she was the first patient he had ever "worked up" all by himself. She feigned surprise and, though too sensitive to be deceived, Bill Michaelson appreciated her friendly attitude.

He finished the lengthy history, began the physical examination and became uncertain and nervous again. Marie was unable to help him with friendly conversation. He did a slow and painstaking physical and laboriously filled in the forms with notes. He called the nurse and probed Marie's pelvic innards in a slow and deliberate manner so forcefully that Marie wondered if he were trying to feel her kidneys through her vagina. Bill apologized for any discomfort he had caused and assured her that he found nothing amiss in her pelvis. He performed a rectal examination, and again Marie had the impression he was really after her kidneys. The intense probing brought on a waves of nausea. Bill was aware that something was wrong as the color had left Marie's face. The nurse brought the requested basin, but Marie did not throw up. Bill apologized for upsetting Marie and left the examining room clearly embarrassed and dissatisfied with his performance. Marie had been too miserable to attempt placating the young man further.

After what seemed to Marie an eternity, Dr. Peter Markley entered the examining room. A distinguished looking man with thick gray hair and moustache, he was efficient and thorough and asked questions of Marie as he quickly examined her body. Within minutes he was through and sat on a stool reviewing Marie's chart. The blood and urine specimens taken on her last visit, three days before, had been analyzed and the results appeared on the variously colored slips of paper, special forms, now attached to the chart. He turned away from Marie who was sitting on the edge of the examining table all vestiges of modesty lost between the flimsy gown and the impersonal prodding and probing entailed in the physical examinations. For several minutes he wrote in her chart, and from what she could see of his face no signs of his usual smile were evident. When he did again turn his attention toward her, she sensed a seriousness in him with which she was unfamiliar.

"Marie," he began. "I hate to frighten you, but I don't like what we're finding. Your blood pressure is rising, your kidney functioning is worsening. We had better admit you to the hospital immediately."

"I can't come in now. Who'll care for the children and Rodney?"

Dr. Markley rose from the stool. "You don't realize the seriousness of this situation. Rodney will have to make arrangements. I want you in now. I'll call Rodney. Do you know his number?" He took the wall phone off the hook and waited.

Marie's head drooped in resignation as she gave Dr. Markley Rodney's phone number, one sign of the gravity of her condition since, in the past she had never called to interrupt Rodney's work. Dr. Markley dialed.

"Rodney? Peter Markley here. I have your wife in the clinic and I would like you to come over." After a moments silence he continued. "Your damn right it's necessary. I wouldn't ask if it weren't. We'll meet in my office in ten minutes." He hung up and his frown slowly turned into that warm smile Marie had found so reassuring in the past. "Get dressed and come up to my office. We'll make arrangements from there. Who's with the kids now?"

"We have a part-time maid. She's with them."

"I think Rodney may be forced to get to know his children," Dr. Markley said with a hint of reproach. Marie, who normally would have bristled, was beyond noticing.

Anticipation filled Jim Kulp as time for the first meeting of the Search Committee approached. He had never before in his academic life been in a position where his decisions affected anyone but himself. Though only one of a six member Search Committee, even wielding a little influence was for him a new experience.

The chairman of the Search Committee was John Block of Medicine. Jim felt he would learn much from observation of the manner in which the committee was managed by that reportedly skilled politician. He was particularly curious about the way in which John would handle Richard Shane of Surgery owing to their similar temperaments and the traditional rivalry between Medicine and Surgery. Both men were ambitious, hard working and rumored to be ruthless when thwarted. John, at forty-nine, was a full Professor and Richard, a thirty-five year old Associate Professor was down one rung on the academic ladder. Both were courted by other schools.

Other members of the Committee were full professors and from non-clinical departments of the basic sciences: Professor Charles Evans of Anatomy and Professor Harry Tatum of Pathology. Professor Lawrence Root of Bacteriology, another basic science, had a joint appointment in Medicine as well.

Jim was the youngest, least experienced and lowest ranking member of the Search Committee.

John Block called the group to order and read a message from the Dean of the Medical School which essentially told them to go out and find a "great" man for the job to spare no effort in convincing him to join the school. This was no small order inasmuch as

Wilder was not in the "Ivy league" and was not even situated in a metropolitan area. Jim had been attracted to the school by the chance to be with Bob Mettlar and liked small town living. Many, he recognized, prefer the excitement of a city and that preference tends to go with the type of person who places great weight in the building of a prestigious reputation. Jim voiced his reservations and was immediately transfixed with less than friendly stares from some on the committee. He had not considered that his remark could be viewed as a slur on their reputation or, as John Block often referred to it, their "national image."

The bulk of the meeting was spent describing procedures to be followed and discussing sources of information regarding possible candidates. It was agreed that a list would be compiled and carefully scrutinized by the committee. Those candidates surviving the culling process would receive a letter of inquiry regarding their desire to be considered for the position. Jim suggested the alternative of ordering the list in descending order, the committee's first choice first, and offering the position to the candidate at the top of the list until one accepted.

"After all," he reasoned, "it is one thing to reject the race and quite another to refuse the prize. We might catch a fish we might never land the other way." His suggestion was completely ignored.

The meeting adjourned after a time had been chosen for regular meetings at two-week intervals. They had met in John Block's office in the Department of Medicine situated on a corridor between the hospital and medical school. Jim walked back to the medical school with Harry Tatum of Pathology.

"It looks like we're in for a long session," Jim said. "We just don't have the bait to catch the sort of fish Dean Mackenzie seems to crave. We're short on space, money and open faculty positions."

"It doesn't look promising," Harry agreed.

"Having Bob Mettlar stay around, though he'd never interfere, would certainly threaten many candidates," Jim admitted. "We'd be smart to choose someone already in the department. What about Rodney Barret?"

"He has a good reputation as a researcher, but I know nothing of his administrative abilities. What about Tony Lewis?" Harry countered.

Jim had forgotten that Harry and Tony were good friends. "I would have no objection to Tony," he said, "but I don't think he rates high with the Dean. His role in bringing the first black student into this medical school saw to that."

Harry smiled thoughtfully remembering how he and Tony led the rancorous fight against the Dean. "We won that battle a few years ago," he said, "but wounds heal slowly. I'll try and find out Frank Mackenzie's feelings, though I suspect your assessment is correct. It's a pity. Tony would make a fine department head and I'm certain he'd like that job."

The two parted and Jim continued to his office where he had an appointment to see a third-year medical student concerning his senior thesis work. At the doorway he was greeted by Donna Beardsley. She had been working for Jim for two years and was to stay for two more until her husband, Andy, graduated. Like many technicians, Donna was the wife of a medical student, and needed employment to help put him through school. An attractive girl, she was also, efficient, talented and friendly. Jim appreciated these attributes and hoped her third-year medical student husband would join the house staff as an intern, climb the residency ladder at Wilder and give Donna more time in his employ.

"Bill Michaelson is waiting in your office," she whispered with raised eyebrows.

"You must have some of the misgivings I do about that young man," Jim lowered his voice. "Do you want me to discourage him from working with us?"

"Can you refuse a student who wants to do a thesis in your field?" she asked in surprise.

"I could try to discourage him if you think I should," he replied.

"Why don't you make the decision," she said.

"You'll be the one training him, working with him, spending time with him. This Search Committee may really cut into my time in the laboratory," Jim said, shaking his head. "A happy technician is a productive technician." He grinned.

"I really don't know him all that well. It's just some things Andy has said." Bill Michaelson and her husband were classmates.

Jim shrugged and entered his office to find Bill sitting behind his desk reading a manuscript Jim had been preparing for possible future publication. Annoyed by Bill's brashness, he endeavored to maintain his poise. He quickly sat down in the chair facing his own desk and trying unsuccessfully to hide the sarcasm in his voice asked, "Do you think it's a good paper, Doctor Michaelson?"

Bill pursed his lips and stared thoughtfully at the desk for what to Jim seemed an eternity. Finally he looked directly at Jim and asked? "Where do you think all that activity is going?"

As that question had been plaguing Jim for the past few months and unanswered represented a weakness which precluded publication, he was grudgingly impressed with this young man's rapid grasp of the material. Jim's annoyance and misgivings lessened as he found himself discussing his work with an intelligent, if somewhat eccentric, medical student.

The misgivings had developed last semester, when Bill, then a second-year student, took the Pharmacology course. Bill received a better than average grade but he appeared unenthusiastic and lazy. Jim was surprised to learn that Bill was on a partial academic scholarship and still lacking the funds necessary to pay for his education, had been "moonlighting". Now the hectic third year schedule made it extremely difficult to find paying work and Bill was getting desperate.

Not only did Jim not discourage Bill from working with him on his senior thesis, he offered him the job of laboratory assistant as his own laboratory dishwasher and animal care helper was about to leave. During the ensuing discussion Bill mentioned that he did not enjoy working with animals as he had a "weak stomach". This prompted Jim to have some second thoughts, but he made it plain that in his job animal care would be a daily requirement. Bill seemed to accept that and their interview was finished.

"I must agree," he told Donna later, "he does seem a little odd, but I sense in him the ability to think and that is rare in students. For that matter, it seems to be rare in faculty as well."

Donna, who was still not sure her boss had made a wise choice, chided him, "Well, well, a thinking dish washer. That's all we need."

"Though it may appear laboratory dish washing's a simple menial chore, it's extremely important. As our analytical methods become more and more sensitive, contamination from inadequate dish washing becomes a serious source for errors."

"That's precisely my point, Dr. Kulp," Donna answered. "We don't need a thinker. We need a worker."

"We'll see. I think he'll work out," Jim replied. "If he doesn't, we can find someone else for the job."

The Hospital Political Affairs Committee met but once a month under usual circumstances. The heterogeneous membership: doctors, nurses, a lawyer, a clergyman, a social worker, made it difficult to find a time when all its members could attend. Furthermore, it was not a group which enjoyed meeting. Despite the euphemistic title, the function of the committee was to designate which patients lacking adequate kidney function would receive the life-prolonging dialyzer treatments and conversely which patients would be condemned to a slow but certain thoroughly unpleasant death.

The crux of the problem was too little money, equipment, and manpower, and too many patients with diseased kidneys. Wilder General Hospital was considered fortunate to have one of the few dialysis units in the area. This, relatively new, technique had been demonstrated to prolong the life of patients with irreversible kidney damage and in some rarer cases even to tide patients over until their kidneys regained normal function.

Dr. Peter Markley headed the dialysis unit, but was not free to choose which patients would receive treatment. He was obliged to call upon this committee for help in such decisions. He called this unusual meeting, the second in September, because he was confronted with a peculiarly delicate emergency situation. The wife of a member of the Medical School faculty had developed complete renal shutdown. He had been dialyzing her on an acute basis. It was now clear that there was little likelihood of renal function recovery, and he wanted to bring her into the chronic kidney program which required decisions from the full committee. Demands exceeded supply.

Marie Barret would soon be dead without dialysis. Rodney Barret's presence on the medical faculty created an uncomfortable situation for Peter Markley and the medical people on the committee.

The Reverend Montrose, hospital Chaplain, inquired, "Do we have the right to give this girl special consideration simply because she is a member of the 'medical family'?"

"We obviously don't, but we will," stormed Jake Bourne, chief of obstetrics. Jake was known for his pragmatism, volatility and lack of sufferance for anything or anybody of whom he disapproved.

"Hold on, Jake," John Block cut in. "We'll consider Marie just as all other candidates for dialysis and then make our decision." What Dr. Block meant was that somehow the committee would assess Marie's contribution to society as compared to the other candidates.

Jake glared at John and restrained his natural instincts though anyone close enough could hear the "bullshit" mumbled under his breath.

"If we put Marie in the program, who goes out?" Hal Smith, the lawyer asked.

"I'm not sure anyone goes out this time," Peter answered. "Mrs. Perez is in terminal coma. A few days more or less can't help her. I recommend giving her place to Marie."

"What will the Perez family's reaction be?" Block asked the social worker.

"It will be a blessing to them," the lawyer cut in, "but a blow to the young man being held for her brutal assault. It now becomes murder."

"Christ!" Jake Bourne exploded. "How complicated can things get? This goddamn committee assignment is the biggest pain in the ass of anything I do."

"Amen," chimed in the Reverend Montrose whose timely sense of humor had proven invaluable to this group many times before.

"I take it that we'll stop dialysis on Perez and arrange for Surgery to put a shunt in Mrs. Barret?" asked nurse Linda Koster who was responsible for the day to day operation of the dialysis unit.

"Not so fast, Linda," cautioned John Block. "We must first get the consensus of the committee."

"Oh hell, John" Jake smirked, "why do you always have to make such a formal deal out of this?"

"You know," admonished Hal Smith. "If ever committee minutes and records needed to be letter perfect, this one's does. And this particular situation is loaded. I don't believe Mrs. Perez's demise is apt to cause us a problem, but how do we justify running Mrs. Barret to the top of the waiting list?"

"The waiting list has rapid turnover," Peter pointed out. "Those who need it most don't stay on it long."

"That, at least, is encouraging," said Jean Tucker, a social worker and the newest member of the committee attending her first meeting.

Jake Bourne stared at her and then broke into a sadistic smile. "Most get off the list by dying, not by getting treatment." he announced.

Miss Tucker paled. "You mean people we could save, die?"

"Every day," Jake said with a shrug, clearly enjoying the effects of apprising this naive social worker of the facts of life and death.

"Why don't we get more machines?" Jean persisted.

"Those we have aren't fully utilized," Jake answered.

Linda Koster turned on Jake. "What do you mean?"

"How many shifts do you run?" he asked.

"Two," she replied.

"So, there are eight hours when the machines aren't being used. The number of dialysis stations isn't the bottleneck. Right?" asked Jake belligerently.

"Jean," Peter Markley explained, we don't have enough staff to man the machines and we don't have the money budgeted to pay extra staff."

"You mean to tell me people die merely for a lack of money?" Jean was incredulous.

"Like flies," Jake bellowed. "Ain't that one hell of a note? We spend all sorts of money on medical research to cure disease and then let people die when there is a cure."

"That's not fair, Jake," John Block calmly asserted. "It's not even accurate. Dialysis is not a cure, it's a crutch, and though it can keep people alive, it is no final answer to the problem of kidney failure. Jean, it's a holding action. Research leading to the cure and prevention of the conditions which cause kidneys to fail is what's needed. In a way, money spent on the crutch takes away from the eventual solution of the problem."

"Tell that to the patient who is living on dialysis," Peter Markley interjected. "I doubt he'd be so altruistic as to agree to turn the paltry sums available to the researchers engaged in kidney research."

This argument was a sensitive one between John Block, an internationally recognized researcher and authority on renal disease, and Peter Markley, the physician who spent his time and efforts treating these patients. Peter invariably lost because John, as head of the Nephrology section of Medicine was his chief, and tended to reward those in his section who were research rather than treatment oriented.

"I was in Washington last week," Hal Smith announced, "and some of you will be happy to know there is legislation brewing which will make money available from the government to defray the cost of dialysis."

"Thank God," said Jean.

"Oh Lord, no!" replied John Block.

"This committee must really confuse the Almighty," the Reverend chimed in.

"Can we get on with it," grunted Jake. "I have happier ways to spend time."

"Besides Marie Barret, we have six other candidates for the open spot," John Block told the committee. "Two we can rule out on age, over fifty, another is diabetic and one, though young and relatively healthy, has been in trouble with the law most of his life. He would contribute problems for society; nothing positive. Here are their charts." He passed them out for the others to scan. "That leaves us Marie and two others whom we could select for dialysis. I don't see how a decision could be made among these three on any rational basis."

For several minutes an uncomfortable silence fell over the room. Each member of the group looked strangely alert. They passed the charts back and forth and read and turned the pages with a grim determination.

John spoke again. "Does anyone differ from my assessment?"

No one spoke.

"Shall we let 'Cavanaugh' decide?"

A murmur of assent arose. "Cavanaugh" was an old warn cardboard hat box with a hole in the top from which names were drawn. John Block wrote on slips of paper while Peter Markley brought "Cavanaugh" from the closet adjoining their meeting room. John folded the papers, placed them in the box and looked at the other committee members.

"Whose turn is it to play God?" he asked.

"I think it's my turn," Peter Markley quietly admitted.

He drew a slip, unfolded it, as a smile brushed his lips, and was missed by no one.

"Marie Barret is to be our next patient," Peter said.

Relief swept the room. Peter and Linda discussed scheduling and the meeting quickly adjourned.

Then John Block did an uncharacteristic thing. Used as he was to positions of leadership, he seldom stooped to menial chores preferring instead to delegate them to others. Today he tidied up the meeting room table and returned "Cavanaugh" to the closet. One might have ascribed his action to a peace offering to the Gods of chance which had just been so obliging. In reality, he wanted to remove and destroy the other two slips of paper bearing Marie Barret's name.

Barely awake at this early hour, Bill Michaelson was changing his clothes for the second time. In the surgical locker room where the male staff and students changed from their street clothes to the apparel worn under the sterile operating gowns, Bill was thinking about the patient he'd "worked up" in the clinic several days before and was, therefore, assigned to accompany into the operating room. It seemed a strange coincidence that she turned out to be Dr. Barret's wife and that he was now working in Barret's department as a dishwasher and laboratory assistant.

The operative procedure entailed placing a tube in her forearm connecting a vein and artery so that access to her bloodstream would be easily available for her thrice-weekly dialyses. Surgically speaking, it was an unexciting procedure and he did not relish the time he had to spend holding retractors or doing whatever "scut work" the surgeons would require of him. In the OR the only thing lower than a medical student was a student nurse. He felt the whole hospital/medical school hierarchy absurd and respected those who treated him as an intellectual equal.

Despite the early hour and his reluctance for the chore at hand, something was making him feel good. Donna Beardsley had turned out to be intelligent and friendly and since he would spend a considerable amount of time working with her he was pleased. He was enjoying the research which was exciting and Donna had suggested that he might enjoy meeting her younger sister who was soon to visit the Wilder campus. It was this prospect that really pleased him. If Donna's sister were as attractive, bright and friendly as Donna, he might really be fortunate. Bill was not very popular and, though he was loath to admit it, he was lonely. He craved female companionship but was too proud and too shy to make the necessary contacts. Donna's captive companionship put him at ease with her. He had little experience with girls, was a virgin and ashamedly believed he was the only one in the medical school. After all, medical students had reputations and all the student nurses were well known to have hot pants.

"Any student here named Michaelson?" called out a young doctor disturbing Bill's reveries.

"Me," Bill signaled.

"I'm Barry Ward," the young surgical resident informed Bill. "You'll be assisting Dick Shane and me placing a Scribner shunt. I hope you're up on the anatomy of the forearm. Shane always asks questions, and if you screw up, he'll pick on me." He grinned at Bill.

"I did some looking last night in 'Cunningham'," Bill answered. "Hadn't opened that book since first year. It even smelled like formaldehyde when I opened it. Funny how that brings back memories."

Barry's locker was near Bill's and he was changing clothes quickly. "I know," he said. "Surgical residents do a lot of dissecting and my wife complains bitterly when I come home. That smell even gets on your breath."

"How long will this take?" Bill asked.

"It isn't a long procedure, but Shane is supposed to be teaching me and the patient being a faculty wife an all, he'll be particularly careful. You know what they say about treating doctor's families. They're always the ones with the complications," Barry said.

"I thought that only applied to MD's. Barret's a Ph.D. isn't he?" Bill asked.

"He's faculty and that's all it takes," Barry explained. "Other patients who develop problems get them taken care of elsewhere so we aren't constantly reminded of our mistakes. If it's in the 'family' you never live it down. Someone ought to do a statistical study and see if there is really anything to the idea that doctors and their families fare poorly in hospitals."

Bill frowned. "It could be," he said "that they're scared silly and don't come to hospitals for trivial reasons and are literally scared to death when they do."

"Could be," Barry agreed. "Let's get moving. Shane won't be happy if we're late."

In the scrub room adjacent to the OR they washed their hands and forearms with a bactericidal soap.

Holding their forearms vertically and dressed in their green scrub suits and hats, they resembled two preying mantises shuffling into the operating suite. The operating room nurses were efficient and businesslike and gowned and gloved the two men. Bill was relieved to have accomplished that step without mishap as there were many stories of the varied ways neophytes manage to break sterility. He stood as far out of the way as possible, a sterile towel covering his gloved hands already uncomfortable from being sheathed in rubber and being clasped and held away from his body in such an unnatural position. Marie Barret was wheeled in and transferred to the table by nurses and orderlies.

"Though this procedure is not difficult it leaves little room for error," Dr. Shane spoke as he entered the OR with nurse Koster and the students and house staff who had come in to observe the procedure. "This patient's condition gives her a tendency toward poor healing and a lessened resistance to bacterial infection. The passages through her skin made by the shunt tubing are invitations to bacterial infection. Thrice weekly manipulations during the attachment and detachment of the dialyzer tubing create potential threats for the introduction of pathogenic bacteria. What is the incidence of infectious complications in these cases?" he asked no one in particular. After a period of silence, he asked, "Whose patient is this?"

Bills hand rose spontaneously. "Mine sir," he answered.

"And whose hand is that risking contamination? Come over to the table and join us, doctor, but please don't touch anything till you get to the sterile area."

Bill picked his way cautiously to the table and wisely kept his distance as the area had not yet been draped with sterile sheets and towels. "I'm Bill Michaelson," he announced.

"Glad you didn't offer to shake hands," Shane observed. There was polite laughter from behind some surgical masks. "Well, Bill, can you answer the question?"

Bill had trouble remembering what was asked and was beginning to panic as he was sure he was about to make some stupid move which would break sterility.

Barry Ward sensed his confusion and whispered, "Incidence of infections?"

"I suspect the incidence of infections must be quite high," Bill answered.

"It is extremely high," Shane said. "Probably close to one hundred percent if the truth were known. We rely on careful sterile manipulations and plentiful cleansing and antibiotics to prevent infection from getting out of hand; but, Dr. Michaelson, are infections the greatest cause of failure for shunts?"

"No, sir" Bill answered, "clotting is."

"I see you have done your homework," Shane replied. "Good! Eventually these shunts clot off and require replacement."

The patient was now draped and the exposed portion of her forearm prepared for the procedure.

"Dr. Ward will do the procedure and I will assist. Miss Koster will assemble the various parts of the shunt and see to it that our placement is proper. Linda knows more about shunts and their care than anyone in this hospital. This patient is unconscious under general anesthesia. Most times we do this under a local anesthesia but as this lady is a faculty wife, the anesthesiologists preferred general anesthesia. Proceed, Dr. Ward, and observe, Dr. Michaelson. I will ask the questions."

"It isn't as though the Dean is always putting you on committees, Jim," Janet Kulp remonstrated. She was trying to sleep after a long day with the kids. She and Jim were in darkness in their double bed and he, unable to sleep, was thinking aloud..

"It's been such a waste of time," he continued, "The rest of the committee act as though I weren't there. Granted I'm the youngest and lowest ranking member, but no one likes being ignored."

"Don't you care who they select? After all he'll be your boss." she asked.

"Of course I care, but I can't see that I'll have much influence on the decision," he complained.

"It's far to early to know that. Give it a chance," she yawned.

"Even my own wife is bored by what I have to say," he sighed.

Janet smiled, "Not what you say, when you say it, Jim. I am so sleepy I am having trouble listening."

Jim turned and kissed her. "Go to sleep Jan."

He lay listening to his wife's rhythmic breathing envious of her drowsiness. His mind wandered the long path which had brought him to his present situation.

His first serious interest in science was sparked by his biology teacher in preparatory school. His plan to major in biology in college, get a graduate degree, and then teach in a preparatory school were interrupted in college by the second world war. Following enlistment and basic training in a medical aid company, he was sent back to college for premedical training and then on to medical school. The war ended during his second year and he was discharged. He decided to take some time off as the accelerated medical school program had been so hectic and obtained a one year instructorship in the Pharmacology department whose course he had just finished.

During that instructorship year he became involved in research and had a taste of the excitement of exploring the unknown in medicine. As a result he decided to get a graduate degree in Pharmacology. He transferred to the department of B. J. Aranow, a renowned pharmacologist in the city where his parents lived.

Dr. Aranow was an exceedingly careful researcher and Jim's time with him helped to make Jim a critical scientist: critical in the sense that he questioned what he read and heard and took little for granted. He also learned to think carefully before he spoke because BJ's favorite question, which stopped many a conversation was, "What is the evidence for that statement?"

Jim took an instructorship in BJ's department to fill the time between finishing his graduate degree and the beginning of the third year of medical school. During that time he met and courted Janet who came to BJ's department as a technician. They were married just prior to his entrance into the third-year medical class.

Toward the end of his senior year Jim was offered an assistant professorship in BJ's department. As both Jim's and Janet's parents lived nearby, Jim decided their marital life might be improved by seeking employment elsewhere. In addition, though flattered by the offer, Jim preferred to get away from BJ who could be difficult. By the simple expedient of confiding his marital/parental problems, Jim was able to enlist BJ's considerable aid in securing employment without seeming to spurn his offer.

BJ learned of an opening in the department of Dr. Robert Mettlar at Wilder University Medical School. Bob was coming north to attend meetings and BJ arranged to have him visit his department and interview Jim regarding possible employment.

As the day for the interview approached, Jim was apprehensive about meeting Professor Mettlar. BJ had assured him that Bob Mettlar was one of the best pharmacologists in the country and that the job in question would be a real opportunity to further Jim's career. BJ had such a "cold" personality that Jim hoped Dr. Mettlar would be more likable.

When they met in BJ's office they sat on the red leather couch facing a bookcase. Jim sat on one end half-turned toward Dr. Mettlar who faced stiffly forward and seemed to be eyeing the titles on the books. Jim was alert and ready to deal with any question Dr. Mettlar might ask of him. He waited for what seemed a long time, his tension growing as the silent moments passed. Dr. Mettlar continued to remain silent. Finally, Jim could stand the silence no longer. "How many members do you have in your department?"

Bob Mettlar seemed to awaken from a trance. "Oh! Dr. Kulp. Two in addition to myself at present." He seemed startled and out of breath.

Jim's nervousness vanished as he realized Bob Mettlar was terribly ill at ease. Jim helped the situation by volunteering answers to questions he felt Bob would have liked to ask under these circumstances. With time Dr. Mettlar relaxed and the two had a long conversation. Jim came to appreciate that under Bob's uneasy exterior there existed a warm and friendly personality which an exquisite shyness shackled. The two men enjoyed each other. They laughed frequently and before the interview was over a visit to Wilder was arranged and a job offer was made and accepted contingent upon Jim's visit with Janet and her concurrence.

Janet's snoring penetrated and interrupted Jim's thoughts and he smiled as he vividly recalled those first painful moments with Bob Mettlar. Now he was a member of a team selected to replace him. He'd have to do a conscientious job no matter how much time it took. His respect, alone, for Bob made that necessary.

"You ready, Mrs. Barret?" the orderly asked. "I'm to take you to the dialysis unit."

Marie slipped from her hospital bed into the wheelchair with help from the practical nurse who had awakened her and given her a sponging just moments before. The fact that she'd had no breakfast did not concern her as she had no appetite. She was constantly thirsty now having been informed by Dr. Peter Markley that she must restrict her fluid intake. She craved, of all things, a beer, a drink she had never coveted.

She looked forward to being dialyzed in the clinic. For one thing, they would be using the week-old shunt in her forearm. All her previous treatments had been accomplished through needles placed in blood vessels in her thighs and these were too close to her private parts for comfort. Though she wasn't a prude, she did not feel comfortable exposed the way she had been. She understood that the troupes of young men and women who marched in and out of her room with their instructors were student doctors and nurses like Bill Michaelson, and she felt guilty resenting them. Somebody has to be used to train neophytes and, though she agreed with the policy at Wilder General Hospital, she couldn't relax. She would be much happier showing her forearm than her bottom. When they arrived at the unit, she was transferred into one of the five lounging chairs placed around the periphery of the room and facing the center. Each of these chairs was part of one dialysis station.

Between the chairs at each station stood a console on wheels resembling a large window air conditioner. These consoles displayed several dials and switches and from them emanated a tangle of plastic tubing. The tubing led to a bath on top of the console which looked like fruit juice dispensers seen continuously stirring in soda fountains and cafeterias.

Marie watched patiently while Linda Koster, using sterile technique, removed the bandages from her forearm to reveal the flexible translucent tubing through which her blood was flowing. The tube, several inches long, formed a "U"-shape with the bottom of the "U" crossing her wrist and the upper ends disappearing into the substance of her forearm where they entered an artery and vein. Marie stared at this arrangement with the distinct impression that it was someone else's arm she was viewing. At the base of the "U" was a connection which allowed the base of the "U" to be parted.

Linda, who was describing each step of the procedure to Marie, cautioned "before opening this connection both sides of the shunt must be clamped closed or else you will lose blood. If ever the clamp opens by mistake, you can pinch the tube closed with your other hand. In an emergency, don't worry about sterility, just stop the blood flow and get help."

Linda connected the individual ends of the shunt to the appropriate plastic tubing of the dialyzer. Marie watched and listened, but it all appeared so complicated and strange she could not imagine understanding or doing the procedure at home as she heard some doctors were recommending. When the hookups were completed, Linda removed her sterile gloves and surgical mask and turned to the console where she began to turn a small dial.

"I am now starting the roller pump which will feed your blood into the tubing to the dialyzer. We'll start priming the blood back through your wrist in a moment. You can see clear solution falling into the basin. That's sterile salt solution which partially filled the system."

When Marie's blood had replaced the saline, Linda clamped the side tube through which the salt solution was dripping into the basin and removed the final clamp from her wrist.

"That's all there is to a hookup," she said with a reassuring smile. "Now sit back and relax and let the machine do the work of your kidneys."

Marie settled back in the chair and closed her eyes thinking she might doze off. It was still early, not yet eight o'clock, and the procedure was causing her no discomfort as had the needles placed in the vessels in her thigh. Sleep would not come and she soon found herself glancing at the TV screen placed in the room to help pass the time. The volume was turned down and she could not tell what the announcer was saying. She began to notice the other patients settling into their stations and was surprised by their youth. At thirty-eight, she was the oldest so far, but then, only three of the five chairs were occupied. The other patients were dressed in street clothes and had come in from outside the hospital. Linda Koster and a young black man were starting the machines for them just as Linda had for Marie, and the two patients were chatting like old friends. They would occasionally glance toward Marie, but a serious perplexed look would appear on their faces when this happened. When all the stations were filled, Marie noted the same behavior from the two newcomers. It seemed like more than the natural shyness people tend to extend toward strangers.

Linda Koster sensed Marie's discomfort and quietly informed her that "Mrs. Perez, whose place you have taken here, was a much loved member of this group. She was the oldest and longest dialyzed member and was a stabilizing influence in times of stress and depression, an example they could look to. Sadly, last week she was senselessly beaten for a few pennies in her purse and isn't expected to survive."

Linda introduced Marie to the group. "We're all going to miss Mrs. Perez," she announced," but she would be the first to want you all to befriend Mrs. Barret, Marie."

"When did she pass?" asked a young black girl.

Linda stared silently at the group for several seconds. "Perez is in deep coma and could die any minute."

"Might not these treatments help her?" was the next question from the group.

"Very unlikely," Linda answered.

"But possible," insisted one of the group.

"Yes it is possible, but it was also certain that Marie Barret would not do well without treatment," Linda said. The four patients were silent and did not allow their eyes to meet Marie's who was astonished at her own boldness in seeking out their glances.

Linda turned to Marie. "This is a fairly usual reaction when the clientele here changes. Each patient feels threatened by newcomers, guilty about being among the chosen, and yet being able to voice these feelings on behalf of other patients without appearing to be self-centered. I encourage the voicing of all sentiments because I believe these thoughts do less harm out than in. Adjustments to be made regarding dialysis are many and not easy. The sooner we make them the better."

Marie closed her eyes and pretended to sleep. Lord, she thought, what have I ever done to deserve this.

Several hundred miles north of Wilder University, in another medical complex sat Sidney Amstel. His small but beautifully appointed corner office in the Pharmacology Department had views of the huge metropolis below. He was staring at the view this

October afternoon, but his thoughts were on the letter he was holding. It was from Dr. John Block of Wilder University Medical School. It informed him of the resignation of Dr. Robert Mettlar as Chairman of Pharmacology, and inquired as to whether he would like to be considered for that position. Sidney was in his early forties and was an associate professor. There was little chance of his becoming chairman of his own department as the incumbent was but two years older than he.

Sidney liked urban life and his wife, a physician, was also on the medical school staff. Sidney was not an M.D., a condition his spouse never let him forget in moments of marital tension. In truth, her reputation was beginning to challenge his own despite his astute political abilities through which he had landed the editorship of a prestigious scientific journal. If he were to become chairman of pharmacology at Wilder, he would automatically be awarded a full professorship, a substantial pay raise, and he would not necessarily have to relinquish the editorship. All these points were attractive.

His research would probably be curtailed by the process of moving and by the numerous details a departmental chairman can attend to, but for sometime his motivation to conduct research had been dwindling. He felt he was a good teacher and he loved teaching. His research was uninspired and was done only because he knew it was expected of him. His writing and organizational abilities had helped make him an editor-in-chief at a very early age. Why should he do research at all? It was absurd, yet he knew he must go through the motions or else be treated as a second-class citizen in the scientific community.

So far, he had managed to carry on a line of research he had started as a graduate student. Then, he had been surrounded by ambitious, able researchers and had done creditable, if undistinguished, work. Now, on his own, he found he had talents in other directions and he preferred to pursue them. Perhaps a chairmanship in this small southern school could be just the answer. It couldn't hurt to look, and he felt his credentials would make him competitive for the position. He would talk it over with Barbara this evening. On second thought, why wait? He began composing a letter.

"Can you see anything?" Impatience and excitement sounded in Jim Kulp's voice as he edged closer to the sink in the dim "safe-light" lit laboratory darkroom where he had come to view the strips of film Bill Michaelson was developing.

"Not yet, Dr. Kulp," Bill replied. "I'm just getting the rack into the developer."

For the past few days they had been trying to find the manner in which their insulin solutions had been losing potency so rapidly. The main object of their present research, to measure the amounts of insulin circulating in the blood of normal and diabetic patients, was hampered by the lack of an appropriate yardstick. The standard known insulin solutions used in their sensitive mouse assay system were proving highly unstable. Without standard solutions containing known concentrations of insulin to compare with the results they obtained with their unknown blood samples, there was no way for them to quantify their results. The instability they had found in their standard solutions was not described in any of the published reports by other workers in this field and Dr. Kulp was perplexed as to why.

He had very recently been able to obtain samples of pig insulin molecules which were tagged with a radioactive iodine atom. Measuring the radioactivity allowed quantitative measurements of that insulin with an ease unobtainable with the mouse assay. With this material, they had confirmed the instability and they were now testing for the possible mechanism of this loss of potency. By simply wrapping the glass containers of radioactive insulin solution with x-ray film, with time, the whereabouts of the radioactive insulin would reveal itself through exposure of the film. The first such experiment had now been completed and only development of the film stood in the way of answers.

"I think I can see an image appearing," Bill announced with excitement.

"Good. At least our exposure was long enough. I was not at all sure it would be," Jim answered with relief.

When enough time elapsed for an image to develop fully, Bill rinsed the film strips in water and placed them in the hypo to fix them permanently. The seconds until they could switch on the light box and view their results passed like minutes. They waited in silence each conscious only of the sounds of their breathing.

When adequate time had elapsed, Bill rinsed the film in water and flipped the light switch on the viewing box. He placed the rack holding the strips against the milky white glass and the men peered intently at the images before them despite the discomfort generated by the sudden brightness.

The strips told a story which came as no great surprise to the men though it was satisfying to have their suspicions confirmed. Insulin is a protein and whenever studied, proteins have been found to stick tenaciously to surfaces. The total amounts which stick are very small; but when, as in this research, they were working with small amounts to begin with, these losses from the solution by sticking to the surface of the container represent sizable proportions of the total.

"That idiot!" Jim exploded.

"Who?" asked Bill, startled.

"R. L. Hanson."

"Isn't he a 'big shot' in the insulin assay field? What's he got to do with this?" Bill asked.

"When I first began this work three years ago, some experiments I did showed this instability. I wrote him then to ask how he made his standard solutions since his publication glossed over that aspect of the work. His answer implied that I must be pretty stupid. He just diluted concentrated solutions down to the desired amount in salt solution. You and I know that doesn't work and now we know why."

"How come he didn't have trouble?" Bill asked.

"I don't know," Jim mused. "Maybe his assay was too insensitive to detect it or the vessels he used didn't absorb insulin, or he knew and was keeping it secret to keep ahead of the field."

"Don't all proteins studied stick to all surfaces?" Bill asked.

"All surfaces studied but not necessarily 'all surfaces'."

"Looks like our work is cut out for us studying surfaces," Bill reflected.

"I guess, but that may lead us too far afield," Jim speculated. "We now know how to prevent the phenomenon. You can see, in that third strip of film, that diluting the insulin in another protein prevents the sticking and that confirms our good assays with the standards diluted in gelatin. I think we should go ahead with them."

"Shouldn't we publish this?" Bill asked.

"You bet. It will make a fine contribution to the field. I just don't understand why someone hasn't published this already," he wondered aloud. Suddenly he thrust his wrist watch toward the viewing box. "Good God! In the excitement I forgot about the meeting. It isn't good for the junior member to come in late even if they don't pay much attention to me." He left the darkroom.

Bill removed the film from the viewing box and returned them to the sink for a more thorough washing. He, too, was late for an appointment. Responsible for closely following Marie Barret's progress, he had discussed her case with Linda Koster of the dialysis unit. Bill was impressed by the rapport Linda had with the patients and the thorough knowledge she had of the complicated procedures and equipment. To learn more about the procedures and some practical aspects of patient management, he had asked Linda for some of her time. Such requests from medical students were rare and Linda could not help being pleased and flattered to be asked to expound on her favorite subject.

He arrived at the unit a few minutes late, but since he was both apologetic and out of breath, Linda refrained from unleashing her widely tasted sarcasm upon him. She spent a good hour demonstrating the equipment, all the while fielding the questions of other nurses, technicians and patients with the ease of a virtuoso. Though she had the reputation of being hard on the medical students assigned to her unit, she had been polite and friendly to Bill. Thus, he was emboldened to suggest that they continue their discussion over beer and pizza at a nearby restaurant that evening and delighted when she accepted his suggestion. He returned to the surgery floor feeling elated as Linda's physical attractions had not gone unnoticed although he realized she was several years his senior.

In the restaurant that evening, he learned that Linda had been involved with dialysis from the beginning of the unit at Wilder some five years previously. He began to have an appreciation for the intense psychological strain that being involved with end-stage renal disease patients can have on those who work with them. As the evening wore on, Linda, who seemed to be unburdening herself as she reviewed the few successfully managed patients and the numbers of complications and lost patients, imbibed white wine slowly but steadily. Bill drank beer and, though he tried to pace himself carefully, by the end of the evening he, too, felt slightly inebriated. They had eaten much and decided a walk might help relieve their feelings of fullness and clear their heads.

The evening was cool as they sauntered dreamily along the myriad of pathways that lined the campus. During their walk Bill tried to explain to Linda the work he was doing with Dr. Kulp and his excitement that afternoon in the darkroom. Linda tried to follow his explanations, but their alcoholic state led to much confusion and laughter and little serious concern for the subject matter.

Suddenly, Bill was tugged toward a small apartment building." This is home," Linda explained. "Care for a nightcap?"

Before he could answer that he had had enough, he found himself inside Linda's apartment with his back to the door which Linda had firmly closed.

"I really should drink coffee," he stammered.

"And spoil this wonderful carefree feeling? Being mentally numb? Not worrying about Mrs. Brown's shunt and Mrs. Smith's libido…?" She turned and faced Bill. "Put your arms around me." It sounded more like an order than the childlike supplication it was. Bill complied but was not prepared for the sudden onslaught that followed. In rapid succession he felt pity, lust, fear, intense excitement and guilt. Linda was at least eight years his senior and though he fantasized similar scenes many times, the reality upset him. He was physically attracted to this woman but he did not want any serious alliance with her and, from his vantage point, things were rapidly getting serious. He could feel the reaction in his groin, and the intense pressure of her body was pleasing and terrifying. In panic, he broke free from her grasp, opened the door and ran into the night.

Back at his room, breathless from the long run he was feeling unsteady from drink, though the encounter with Linda had done much to sober him. He lay on his bed wide awake, sleep a seeming impossibility. He felt embarrassed and assumed he had just blown an excellent chance to lose his virginity with a highly desirable woman. Why had he run? He recalled something someone had once told him. "If a woman wants it and you won't comply, you're a damned coward!" If his classmates were ever to learn of this, he'd die. He didn't think Linda would tell. Oh hell! How can I face her, he thought.

Thus tormented, he lay for what seemed an eternity. Slowly he calmed down. He concluded that sex for him could never be casual. Love for his sexual partner had been inculcated into his being by conservative parents from an early age. Though there were times, such as tonight, he wished he could shake off his conscience, he felt the price he would pay would outweigh any temporary pleasures. Thus resigned, he finally relaxed and drifted off to sleep.

Early next morning, Linda Koster sat opposite Peter Markley in Peter's office. As they tried to do at least once weekly, they were reviewing the patients on dialysis.

"I heard Mrs. Perez died last night," Peter began.

"She hung on surprisingly long without dialysis," Linda observed, "but she never regained consciousness. She was our prize patient, a real rock. We needed her example for the younger patients, …gave them the guts to go on. And some lousy creep has to mug her. It isn't fair."

"I know, Linda, it's damn discouraging. How will the other patients respond to that news?"

"Not well. It will be awful on the unit."

"At least she didn't die from her disease. Well, not as a primary cause," he corrected himself.

"That's not important, Peter. You know how fragile their morale is."

"What's the reaction to Marie Barret?"

"What you'd expect. Not good. I think she's tough enough to withstand it. As she's older than the rest I've been counting on her to take Perez's place as their mother figure."

Peter shook his head. "It's strange. No matter how you figure, it's impossible to predict who'll do well and who'll do badly on this therapy. I don't know what the difference is or how to go about finding out."

"What about lab data?" Linda asked.

"That reflects conditions when it's grossly changed but by then you can look at the patient from across the room and tell he's sick. As to fine tuning with laboratory data, every year at the Nephrology meetings someone comes up with a new approach and we all get excited for a time, but it doesn't last. We don't even know what to measure."

"What about renal toxins?"

"What about them? Same thing; every year new ones are discovered and a new bandwagon forms which has its supporters and detractors. Hell, if I choked off the sewer in front of your house, what value would it have to study the pile-up for a few isolated ingredients that caused the smell? All that crap smells. You have to get rid of it all."

"That's what we're doing with dialysis. Isn't it" Linda asked.

"Yes, that's true; but we still don't know what we're doing."

"Hell, Peter, you can't have it both ways. You can't put down research and complain of ignorance."

"You're right. I guess this is why John Block really isn't interested in dialysis. He knows it's just a holding treatment. The better approach would be to avoid kidney failure or reverse it. But someone has to do this. We can't just let them die when simple filtration with that cellophane membrane can sustain life."

"What kind of a life? That's the problem," Linda said and then added, "I think most patients prefer a life on dialysis to the alternative. Though it can get pretty discouraging watching them."

"Any problems other than those Mrs. Perez's death will cause?" Peter asked.

"We're running low on blood to prime the cellophane coils but the blood bank has put out an emergency plea and if we get the usual response we'll be ok."

"You watch, if the government begins to fund this field, industry will come up with commercial dialyzers which won't need so much priming volume and the blood problem will vanish."

"I wish they'd hurry up.," Linda said. "Blood priming makes the whole procedure laborious. Wouldn't it be great to avoid that?"

"We could avoid it now if we used Keil boards."

"Then we'd be stuck with cleaning them between runs. At least the coils are disposable."

"I guess it depends where you want to put your efforts," Peter concluded. "Any problems with your help?" he asked.

"Only the usual gripes about scheduling but, in general they're pretty good. Got a lot of unusual interest from one kid in medical school. Marie Barret is his patient, and he seems genuinely interested in learning about the technology."

"That is unusual," Peter remarked, "but why would you refer to a medical student as a 'kid'? You're not that ancient."

"Believe me, Peter, he's a kid, but a bright one," Linda answered with a smile.

They discussed the individual patients in detail. When it came to Marie Barret, Linda noted she was making progress and seemed to be adapting, but that her husband did not appear to be supplying as much support as he might. Peter was aware of this and suggested Linda have a talk with Rodney.

When they had finished their discussion, Peter asked, "Is there anything unusual troubling you, Linda?"

"No. Why do you ask?"

"You seem more subdued than I've ever known you to be."

"Perez has me down. I'll snap out of it, Peter, don't worry."

Peter Markley did worry. He had seen the signs of discontent in dialysis personnel before. He well appreciated the emotional demands upon such help, and he was firmly convinced there was just so much of this type of service a given individual could endure.

Dean Mackenzie sat at his desk facing the entrance to his office. His visitor, Terry Brown, stood hesitantly in the doorway intimidated by, among other things, a large confederate flag covering the wall behind the Dean's back. This visit was occasioned by a poor grade Terry had made in his first biochemistry examination and he was an out of state student and a "Yankee" to boot. Though his father was a classmate of Frank Mackenzie's at a northern medical school and that had led to his applying to Wilder, he was not at ease with the austere Dean.

"Come in, Terry," Frank Mackenzie coaxed. "Sit down."

"Yes, sir."

The Dean eyed the contents of an open folder before him. "You are not doing well academically. What's the trouble?"

"Biochemistry," Terry croaked. He cleared his throat. "I find it hard. Chemistry is like Greek to me."

"I'm acquainted with that problem," the Dean sympathized, "but you will have to bring that grade up if you want to continue your course of study. Are you putting enough effort into your work?"

"The results wouldn't suggest that, sir."

"I called you in because I want to warn you before you fail. If you already know you must work harder then perhaps this conversation is superfluous." The Dean stared silently at Terry and then asked, "Are you enjoying medical school?"

"Except for doing badly, yes."

"I want to be certain medicine is something you yourself want and not a career foisted on you by a doctor parent. Such pressuring does occur and may not always be apparent to admission committees. The result may be much unhappiness and time wasted."

"No sir, Dean Mackenzie, I do want to become a physician even if I have to learn biochemistry to become one."

"Good, can I help?"

"Can you tutor me in biochem?"

"Lord no! That field has grown so since your dad and I were in school."

"Does a physician really need to know all that material to practice medicine?"

Dean Mackenzie looked sharply at the student before him. A slight smile crossed his usually dour, poker face. It then vanished. "Raise that grade," he demanded. "Make sure the confidence the admissions committee and I have placed in you is justified. Next semester you'll be taking Pharmacology and Pathology. Each of those will require a lot of effort. If you haven't been working hard enough, you had best get started and stay in the habit."

"Yes, sir," said Terry and started rising to leave. At that moment a secretary entered the room.

"I'm sorry to interrupt you, sir, but Dr. Block would like a word with you if possible," she said.

"It's all right, Jenny, our talk is finished." He dismissed Terry with a nod of the head. "Come in, John," he called through the open door. Jenny and Terry stepped aside to let Dr. Block enter, and then left closing the door behind them.

"How goes it, John?"

"Fine, Frank. I wanted to firm up some dates with you. Trying to combine the schedules of several people is almost impossible. Dr. Sidney Amstel, a candidate for the Chairmanship of Pharmacology is able to visit us next week and I wondered if we could set up appointments with you now. If his visit can't be next week it will be some time before I can assemble the appropriate people."

The Dean consulted his calendar. "I'll make time next week. I want this settled as soon as possible. There are several other appointments coming up soon and I consider this one key—of the utmost importance."

"You realize, we don't have a great deal of inducement…"

The Dean cut in. "Damn it John! Don't give me excuses. We have a fine school in a beautiful location. The 'southern part of heaven' it has been called. Anyone we would care to have must appreciate that. This school has a fine reputation and is in a growing phase. Any industrious and ambitious scientist with an ounce of vision ought to recognize the great potential this position affords to build a fine department."

John Block knew better than to argue with Dean Mackenzie when he was extolling the virtues of his school. "Yes sir. I was referring to the limited space and the former head's continued presence."

The Dean's manner changed abruptly. "We may be able to squeeze out some more space, but I don't know what we can do about Bob Mettlar. The lifetime salary support he gets from his career investigatorship leaves me little leverage," he mused. "He brings in sizable amounts of research monies so I can't take his space. He could leave and go elsewhere, and there are many schools that would be delighted to have him. The positive attributes so far outweigh the problems he presents me." He glanced at John Block and added, "I take it he is not one of your favorites?"

"Do you realize that man accused me of lying? I have that in a letter from him." John Block's face had reddened.

The Dean smiled another of his rare smiles. "Oh, John. You can cope with Bob. He does try to act as the conscience of this school at times and that can be inconvenient."

John, upset by his thoughts, had almost forgotten one purpose of his visit. "Oh yes, Frank, I wondered whether you and Millie could come to dinner next Thursday evening. Dr. Amstel and some of the committee will be there."

"I'll check and let you know but I'm reasonably certain we can make it. You getting any reaction from the Pharmacology Department concerning possible candidates?"

"Not much. It seems Jim Kulp knows Sidney Amstel better than anyone else in this school. They were members of the same department. Jim did not suggest him. I asked why and Jim said he'd just didn't think of him but he did not seem to have anything against him. Jim prefers Rodney Barret because he says he's the best qualified of the insiders and the lack of inducements for outsiders dictates…" John's voice trailed off as he realized from the Dean's demeanor that his utterance was unacceptable.

The Dean leaned back in his chair and stared at the ceiling. Despite his nearing retirement age he was an extremely forceful figure. He closed his eyes and for a moment John thought he had fallen asleep though the tautness of his neck and jaw muscles belied that thought. Finally he whispered, "John, don't let Rodney get that appointment."

Dr. Block could barely hear the words, but their intensity left little room for doubt and none for questions. The meeting was over.

The clear blue sky was losing its intensity in the rays of the setting sun. November's cool air was delightful and supportive of Bill's feelings of excitement as he briskly walked toward the Beardsley's modest apartment in one of the revamped army barracks which littered so many campuses following the second world war. He walked because it was close and because he did not own a car.

A rarity among his peers, paying his own way, unmarried, serious about his work, Bill was viewed as a "loner" by the rest of his classmates, and had no close friends. The need to support himself was partially responsible. He felt fortunate to have landed the job in Dr. Kulp's laboratory. It fit his needs and scheduling problems perfectly, he liked the work and he was comfortable with Donna. He was happier than he could ever remember being. *Perhaps I'm not the "melancholy Dane" my mother accuses me of being*, he thought.

He prayed he would find Donna's sister as likable as Donna, though, until this moment, he had not thought about spending an evening with Andy Beardsley whom he had known only casually in their two years together as medical students. He emerged from a passageway between two barracks and saw Andy, fanning the blaze in a charcoal barbecue, behind a wire fence which enclosed the Beardsley's back yard. Andy looked up as he drew near.

"Hi, Bill, come through the gate down there," Andy shouted. "How's surgery treating you?" Andy was on Obstetrics and all students were hungry for any information concerning the various clinical clerkships they had yet to encounter.

"So far so good. They keep us busy: histories, physicals on new patients, holding retractors in the OR. I sleep well at night when I'm not called to emergency surgery. Wish we didn't have so many blood counts, urinalyses and IV's to start. I really need more time to read in the library."

Andy nodded. "I know," he agreed. "Just when we're really motivated to study, they pile on the 'scut work' and we can't. It's stupid."

"Always bitching, you two!" Donna appeared carrying a tray of food.

"Let me help you," Bill offered.

Donna had already deposited the tray on a picnic table.

"Marian will be out shortly," she announced. "Help yourself to a beer, Bill" she motioned to an ice chest under the picnic table. "Did you get to that pile of beakers I left in the sink? Sorry about that, but they seem to pile up by the end of a week."

"No problem," Bill replied. "They're in the drying oven now. I even finished them in time to do some reading. I've got some ideas for experiments on this adsorption thing."

"Are you characters going to waste this evening talking shop?" Andy asked.

"It's just a question of which shop we talk about, love, the clinic or research," Donna answered.

"I'll be lost in either case," Marian Marsh, Donna's sister announced as she joined the threesome.

"Marian, this is Bill," Donna said.

Bill shook Marian's extended hand and was immediately captivated by the directness of her manner and the warmth of her demeanor. Though, physically, she did not resemble Donna, she was a very attractive girl. Smaller, though well proportioned, the combination of black hair, blue eyes and a pale white skin without blemish was striking. Bill's fear of disappointment on finally meeting Marian were dispelled. She was intelligent, friendly and very easy to talk to. The evening passed rapidly and by the time it ended, Bill knew he must see more of Marian.

"Will you be staying long?" he asked.

"Just for the weekend. Then I go back to school in the mountains," she answered. "Donna's been encouraging me to transfer here for ages."

Andy smiled, "She's really out to get some cheap baby sitting," he said.

Bill looked perplexed not realizing the Beardsleys had a child.

"Our little one is only six months old. She doesn't make much fuss in the evening, but you should hear her in the early morning," Donna added.

"I'll take that hint," Bill said. "It is getting late."

"I didn't mean that as a hint," Donna insisted.

"The hell you say," her husband replied with a broad smile.

On his walk home, Bill's mood was far better than could be explained by the alcohol he had imbibed. He was charmed by Marian. He found it odd that in his fantasies he could imagine sexually ravishing a prospective unseen date; yet, once he'd met her face-to-face his fantasies were never erotic if he truly liked her. Following the encounter with Linda Koster he had begun to wonder whether he was normal. Could he enter into a sexual relationship with anyone? He forced these thoughts from him as he could feel his joyous state of mind beginning to slip. He hurried toward his room in the small boardinghouse near the hospital trying furiously to think of a logical reason to call on the Beardsleys the next day before Marian left. Why hadn't he asked her to do something with him on Sunday? It was too late to call now. Oh hell, he thought, why am I so dumb?

Meanwhile, Donna, Marian and Andy had cleaned up the evening's debris and retired. Andy was snoring following a love-making session which, though satisfactory, suggested to Donna a degree of preoccupation which for Andy was quite out of the ordinary. Something seriously troubled her husband. She noticed him to be uncharacteristically subdued during the evening, and assumed him to be uncomfortable in Bill's presence. When asked, he denied not liking Bill and went further to suggest approval of an alliance between Marian and Bill should one develop. Donna was bewildered. It was unlike her husband to keep anything from her.

As he often did, Rodney Barret spent the greater part of the day in his laboratory. He ate supper in the hospital cafeteria and went back to his office to catch up on overdue correspondence. Before Marie's illness, he enjoyed working long hours. Though he suspected a more efficient person could accomplish as much as he in a shorter time, he was friendly and gregarious and spent much time in conversation with his staff of technicians, post doctoral assistants and medical students when their course was in session. Through this daily contact he kept close contact on the progress of his research and teaching. Rodney's obvious diligence stimulated his staff and with their help he was able to accomplish Herculean tasks in his chosen field of research which demanded great effort to produce worthwhile results.

Now that Marie was ailing, slivers of guilt impinged upon Rodney's enjoyment of his efforts. Couldn't he write letters as well at home? Why didn't he spend more time with Marie? These questions did not come from Marie. She had always put Rodney's work first. She had never complained and was not doing so now. Dr. Peter Markley had done it, but Rodney was aware that Marie had not put him up to it and would have been upset had she known.

Peter spent time informing Rodney of the depressing details of what he might expect from Marie's illness. He described the range of possibilities from a rapid downhill fatal course to a longer life tied thrice weekly to dialysis treatments. He alluded to the possibility of a truly normal life following a kidney transplant, but included all the difficulties involved and the lack of long-term experience with that procedure. He emphasized the effects of the illness on Marie's psyche and her need for Rodney's support. Rodney had thanked Peter and then tried to push the conversation from his mind and pretend nothing had changed. Because he was a kind person and because seeing Marie, one could not dismiss her condition easily, dissatisfaction with himself was slowly penetrating his being and causing him to worry—an unusual activity for Rodney.

Another facet of Marie's illness was affecting Rodney. Her sexual desire had vanished. Rodney enjoyed sex; but in the past, owing to his dedication to work, it had been less important to him than to Marie. Now that the tables were turned, he did not like having his advances rebuffed and he felt guilty imposing his desires on an unresponsive partner. In the past, his wife's satiation had required all his available energies and any attention he received from female acquaintances he could easily ignore. Now, temptations were arising where they had not previously. Natural caution and the realization that scandal might hurt his chances for the departmental chairmanship, which he felt was now a possibility, dictated that he reject any sexual favors he was offered.

A knock on his office door startled him as his staff had long since departed.

"Come in," he shouted.

When the door opened, he recognized Linda Koster. In his present confused state her pleasing appearance actually prompted a racing of his pulse. He wondered how she managed to look so desirable at the end of her long working day.

"I couldn't help seeing you in the cafeteria tonight," she started, "I hope you won't resent my butting in, but I want to speak with you about Marie."

Rodney rose and motioned her to a seat but said nothing.

"I'll be direct," Dr. Barret," your wife is adjusting badly to her problems, and I feel you are largely to blame."

"In what way?" Rodney asked, but he did not feel the displeasure he tried to put into his voice.

"My job brings me into very close contact with a small number of patients," Linda began. "To suggest that I not become emotionally involved with them, is absurd. If I didn't care, I doubt I could help them. Aside from the technology, I spend my efforts trying to promote as happy a state of mind as is possible under trying circumstances. How successful I am, is dependent upon the patient. In Marie, I sense a strong personality momentarily lost, too proud to scream for the help she desperately needs. I don't ordinarily seek out spouses. They usually come to me in the normal course of treatments or we send out a social worker. I assume you'd prefer a direct contact and took this opportunity."

"Of course. I'm glad you've come."

"I realize, too, that husbands, wives, families of end-stage renal disease patients have adjustment problems."

Rodney was struck by the term "end-stage."

Linda went on. "If I can help my patients and their families adjust to the realities of the situation, the whole process seems to go more smoothly. Unhappy patients can disrupt my whole unit and damage a very fragile morale."

Rodney noted the fiercely possessive attitude Linda was voicing about the dialysis unit and she must have too because she then she said, "My job can't be done in a half-committed way. If I come on strong, it's because the problems are too depressing to battle halfheartedly. When I chastise you for not supporting your wife it's partly because I believe it's an accurate assessment of the situation and partly because it relieves some of my frustrations at not being able to help my patients live happier lives." Linda paused and the volume in her voice dropped. "I don't usually get this emotional, but I don't usually have faculty wives as patients, nor access to their husbands at the end of a long day. I'm sorry."

Rodney sighed. "Don't apologize, Linda. Your assessment is on target. Between Marie's reticence to accept support and my resentment at having my nice, neat world disrupted, we haven't faced reality, preferring it would go way. What do you suggest?"

"First, give her more time. If you love her, face the fact that your time together may be shorter than you imagined. Enjoy your children together and you must take more responsibility for them. You could soon be their only parent. They, too, need you. The entire family's security has been threatened. You must shore it up. I sense Marie has been their strength in the past. Now she needs that strength for her own support. You must support your children. If she sees this happening, she'll relax her fears concerning how her family's future will be without her."

"Won't that take away her will to fight this thing?"

"I don't think so. It is more likely to decrease her concerns and help her adjust. Though I can't prove it, I have the impression that it's the contented cows in my herd who fare best. Besides, you owe that to your children."

Rodney found that this intense female lecturing him reminded him of his mother and was surprised that he did not resent it. Instead, he found it strangely titillating and was immediately ashamed of the involuntary reaction taking place in his loin.

"Marie comes to my unit early tomorrow morning. Why not come with her?" Linda asked. "Learn the techniques so you can help. You might even elect to treat her at home. Some do well on home dialysis, and it seems especially appropriate in your case."

"I'm not a physician, Linda."

"No, but you are laboratory oriented and you're not squeamish."

"I'm not so sure about that. Animals and humans aren't the same."

"We don't have to make decisions quickly." She sat up straight. "Will you come?"

"I have a nine o'clock appointment, but I'll bring Marie in and stay for a while."

"Thank you, Dr. Barret. I don't think you'll be sorry." She paused then rose from her chair. "Ignore any objections Marie may have. She needs your help very much." Linda Koster walked to the door and was gone before Rodney had managed to rise from behind his desk.

"I'll see you in the morning, then," he announced to no one in particular.

Sunday morning early Bill was passing the street where the Beardsley's lived on his way to the lab to check on Dr. Kulp's experimental animals. On impulse, he turned down the street hoping for a chance meeting with Marian. He was rewarded to find Donna and Marian in the front yard playing with the Beardsley child. They hailed him as he was passing, and it was decided he would show Marian around the laboratory.

At first, he was nervous and ill at ease alone with Marian; but his familiarity with the surroundings and Marian's genuine interest in what he was showing her, energized his self-confidence and allowed his enthusiasm for his work to become apparent. He patiently explained the problems they were trying to solve.

Marian was intrigued by the row upon row of mouse cages which to her resembled library stacks. Bill explained how these mice were used as the basis for a sensitive test for insulin by the simple expedient of injecting them and following their blood sugar response. Their sensitivity to insulin was increased by removing their pituitary and adrenal glands and rendering them diabetic by giving them alloxan, a chemical that destroys the cells which produce insulin. Such mice require special care and are extremely sensitive to minor environmental changes. They had to be kept in a special area in Dr. Kulp's laboratory rather than being housed upstairs in the general animal quarters. These details clearly fascinated Marian and Bill enjoyed relating them.

When the time came for Bill to check up on the dogs in the upstairs quarters, he seemed reluctant to have Marian accompany him. She insisted that she see it all.

"Okay," he said,"but the smell up there is pretty bad."

The elevator stopped at the top floor and they got off and Marian was struck by the acrid, pungent odor which immediately assailed her nostrils. Bill abruptly strode off and disappeared into a room on the left of the hall. Surprised, Marian followed in time to see Bill vomiting into a sink. He straightened up, turned on the taps and wiped his mouth on a paper towel.

"This is the only part of this job I hate," he said clearly embarrassed.

"Are you ill?" she asked in confusion.

"I do this every time I come up here," he answered. "That damn smell gets to me. The first time I get it every day, I retch. Funny, the mouse smell doesn't bother me, but this dog smell does."

"That happens regularly?" She seemed incredulous.

He nodded.

"Does your boss know?" she asked.

"I alluded to my 'weak stomach' for animal work when I signed on, but it's part of the job." He shrugged. "This is why I didn't want you up here," he confessed.

Marian was quiet. She spoke no more while they were in the animal quarters hoping to shorten their stay there. Bill, misunderstanding her silence, felt it signified a dislike of him. He, too, became quiet and the friendly rapport which had grown so rapidly seemed to vanish.

Bill hurriedly finished his work and almost wordlessly walked Marian back to the Beardsleys. At the gate to the yard, Marian asked Bill in; but he declined, unsure of the sincerity of her invitation. He said goodbye and hurriedly left. Marian, who would have truly liked his company, shrugged and went inside.

"Do you realize he throws up each time he goes to the animal quarters?" she asked Donna when reporting on her tour.

"He mentioned something about a weak stomach when he was hired, but Dr. Kulp thought he was trying to get out of work. We now know that's not Bill's style, but I didn't realize he actually vomits when he goes upstairs." Donna was visibly surprised.

"He seemed upset to have me present."

Donna smiled. "He likes you and probably felt it wasn't manly."

"Nonsense, he can't be that dumb."

"Bill has some pretty old fashioned ideas, especially about males and females. How did you enjoy the tour otherwise?"

"Fascinating, I envy you your work. It's like a treasure hunt," Marian said.

"Yes it is," her sister replied thoughtfully. "Despite the routine, every day is different. The mouse assays are slow and tedious but each day's results helps to build a story. There are times when nothing seems to go right and you feel like you are backsliding and then something happens to let you know you are on track again and making progress toward your goal. That's a wonderful feeling and makes everything else worthwhile. It's exciting knowing you're treading ground no one else has ever tread. Probing the unknown." Suddenly Donna's face flushed. She smiled self-consciously, "Pretty heady stuff," she admitted." You must think me nutty."

"Not at all. I envy you. Really I do."

"Then transfer here. You could major in some science, find a job like mine."

"Tempting thought," Marian replied, "I'll give it serious consideration."

"Who's up for the next patient?" asked Andy Beardsley, seated in the nurses' station of the Obstetrics/Gynecology ward reviewing charts. This was Thursday afternoon and Friday mornings Dr. Jake Bourne, Chief of Obstetrics/Gynecology, held student rounds. Andy was one of the students left who had not yet presented to Jake and he was searching through his patient's charts for one whose case would make a good presentation. It was said that this presentation to Jake was largely responsible for the grade third year students would receive in Obstetrics. Andy planned to spend the evening preparing, if he could ever decide which patient to present. The case had to be given from memory as Jake would not allow the students to consult notes during the presentation. Andy hoped he would not have to work up a new patient as that would interfere with his study time. As no one answered, he again asked, "Who in hell is up for the next patient?"

Without looking up from his reading a slightly built young man answered, "Beardsley, why don't you get off your ass and look on the bulletin board?"

Andy sprung from his seat and grabbed the young man by the shirt front.

"You son of a bitch," he shouted, "be civil when I ask a question!"

The young man yelled back, "What in hell's your problem, Andy? You're so damned jumpy lately."

Andy loosened his hold on the smaller man and ashamed said, "Sorry, Fred, guess I'm overtired. All these late night deliveries. They are beginning to wear me down. Doesn't anyone know whose up next?" They all responded rapidly, but no one did.

He walked out of the nurse's station to the hall bulletin board and was relieved to find his name was not at the top of the list which would probably assure him of an evening off to prepare for the next day's presentation. Returning to the nurse's station, he continued his chart review. His difficulty was that the case he felt would make the most interesting presentation and which he knew best, had been a forceps delivery he had attended two evenings before. The delivery, long and difficult had caused certain complications and would make for good discussion. In the chart, however, there was no mention of the use of the metal forceps during the delivery. The resident's notes clearly stated the case as a normal spontaneous delivery. Though tired, Andy was certain he was not confused about what he had witnessed. When the resident who had delivered the baby came into the nurse's station, Andy hailed him.

"Dr. Willis," he asked, "Is there some mistake here?" He held out the chart in question. "Wasn't this a forceps delivery?"

Dr. Willis glanced at the chart, moved close to Andy, and speaking quietly said, "Dr. Bourne has been getting on us for being too free with the forceps. This way we have fewer forceps deliveries, and everyone is happy." He winked conspiratorially and left.

I'll be damned, thought Andy. Hospital charts are supposed to be accurate documents. Hell, I can't present this case.

He spent the next hour finding another case and getting angrier by the minute. This place is supposed to be a teaching hospital, he reasoned. What must go on in non-teaching institutions where no one keeps tabs on the doctors! His thoughts suddenly jumped to another incident which he had witnessed earlier in his clinical clerkship and he visibly shuddered.

The studies of insulin adsorption to surfaces had begun to bear fruit and Jim was excited. With the help of his two assistants, enough experiments had been performed to allow him to write up the work in what he considered a publishable form. The completed manuscript had been sent off to a journal. At the same time, he had sent a copy to Dr. Jean Bower at the National Institutes of Health in Bethesda, Maryland. Jean was a pioneer in the micro-insulin assay field and had been helpful when Jim had started this line of research several years ago. He was pleased to find that her response contained an invitation to be a participant in a small conference to be held at the Institutes for the purpose of discussing the assay of insulin in blood. As few were working in this field, and they were spread worldwide, this government-sponsored meeting would bring together workers who might never meet under ordinary circumstances. This opportunity was one he could not miss. As the meeting was to take place only a day's drive from Wilder, he planned to combine the trip with a weekend in Washington for Janet and himself. Fortunate to be able to get his parents to baby-sit, he and Janet looked forward to the trip and a respite from the usual routine.

Jim had reviewed the original manuscript with Bob Mettlar and following several lengthy sessions had come up with a final version which left no room for doubt concerning exactly what he had done.

"A good paper," Bob repeated over and over again, "is one which a worker in your field can repeat from your written instructions and obtain the same results." Jim was painfully aware there were all too few of these in the medical literature.

Having undergone Bob's rigorous scrutiny, he had little doubt of the validity of his work. He was, nevertheless, nervous as he had almost no experience delivering a paper before a group of his peers. He had no idea of how he would perform. He planned to read his talk as the time he had been allotted was short, and he did not want to leave out any important information. Janet, too was nervous, and it was agreed that she would not attend the meeting, but would instead take advantage of the time to sleep late and do some Christmas shopping in Washington.

Jim's portion of the conference was delivered early in the day. When he finished, there were no questions nor discussion of his results. It seemed as though no one had even heard him give the talk. His work was totally ignored and he was thoroughly depressed.

Driving back to the hotel following the day's scientific activities, one observer of the conference who was riding with him said, "You certainly threw a wet blanket on that conference." Until that moment

Jim had been too emotionally concerned with what he perceived as his personal failure, to recognize the reality of the response to his talk. He, a relative newcomer to the field, had caste serious doubt on the validity of much of the work so far done in the field. He was suggesting that the yardstick used to measure insulin in body fluids was faulty and, therefore, the measurements themselves were faulty. Even more disturbing was the idea that the insulin activity some investigators had found in blood might have arrived there from the surfaces of vessels into which the blood had been collected rather than from within the body from which the blood had been taken.

That evening Jim and Janet took some of the foreign visitors for a tour of Washington. A November summer-like evening, the ride around the various national memorials and government buildings made for a lovely experience and helped to elevate Jim's mood. Returning to the hotel, they all stopped at the bar for a night cap, promised to correspond on their latest work, and planned to visit each other's laboratories should further opportunities for foreign travel arise.

Back in their room Janet asked, "Others from Wilder have gone to Europe on sabbaticals, why not the Kulps?"

"If we can keep our work going and get out some good publications, perhaps we can," Jim speculated.

To Janet, he didn't sound very assured. "Certain members of our Wilder faculty are often on jaunts to fascinating places," she observed.

"I've noticed that too," he agreed, "and should an opportunity to further my research require such travel,

I would be more than willing; but I won't cook up a trip with research as an excuse."

There followed one of those futile husband/wife arguments which serve to blow off pent-up steam and, in this case, sent each partner off to a separate single bed.

"We get so little time to ourselves, it seems criminal to waste it in single beds," he announced to the surrounding room.

"Humph," was the only reply he heard from the other bed.

At some point during the night, reason or hormones must have prevailed, for the early morning sunlight pierced a slight crack in the drawn window curtains and fell on a pair of men's pajama pants lying on the floor in front of an empty bed.

Donna Beardsley and Bill Michaelson were sitting in Dr. Kulp's office proofreading a manuscript. Donna was reading aloud from the newly typed version of their first paper which had been rejected. Bill was following her progress on the marked up copy. When she had finished, Bill shook his head slowly. "You'd think we were trying to push a new and unproven cure for cancer from the troubles we're having getting this simple phenomenon accepted for publication." He was referring to the binding of small quantities of insulin to the surfaces of containers with insulin in them unprotected by the presence of other proteins.

"Since his talk at the NIH meeting, Dr. Kulp thinks this paper is threatening to the leaders in this field who seem to have been unaware of the existence of this phenomenon, or at least haven't mentioned it in their publications. I find it difficult to understand how they missed it."

"I can see how it was missed," Bill answered. "The assays for such small amounts are far from precise, and they probably worked with freshly diluted standard solutions where the losses are less striking. Dr. Kulp stumbled on it because he used a very sensitive assay. It wasn't till we worked with the radioactively labeled insulin that we were certain it occurred. What I don't understand is, now that our data clearly show the phenomenon, why we can't get it published. The same phenomenon occurs with many other proteins. There are publications on those. Why not insulin?"

Jim Kulp had entered his office in time to hear Bill's last remarks.

"I think," he answered, "the problem is that the adsorption of proteins to surfaces has been studied mostly by the biophysicists as a general phenomenon. In terms of absolute amounts lost, so little protein is involved that there has not been much practical significance to the phenomenon. In this situation where we are trying to measure the very small normal amounts in circulating blood, the phenomena of these losses begins to take on a new and very real significance."

"But in view of that very fact, why are we having trouble getting this published?" persisted Donna.

"Now you are probing into one of my pet peeves," he answered. "When a manuscript comes to a journal, the editor-in-chief selects reviewers to look it over. These reviewers are usually well established investigators who have published in the field with which the manuscript deals. They're usually individuals who have been responsible for the direction a field has taken. If the manuscript contains new ideas or data critical of the earlier work, the inevitable happens. You hear so much about scientific objectivity, but our system of manuscript review neither fosters nor demonstrates it. Reviewers are usually kept anonymous which seems to be a further license to subjectivity and irresponsibility.

"I'll bet the reviewers for this manuscript are investigators who were unaware their insulin standards were faulty and that what they measured in blood may have come from the surfaces of improperly washed glassware. This a threat to the validity of their work. They're embarrassed and perhaps subconsciously wish to delay or prevent publication. As you can see from the remarks the editor sent us with the rejection, he's completely missed the point. He suggests sending the paper to a pharmacy journal as he thinks the producers of insulin will be interested in the losses on the insulin vials used for treating diabetics. The percentage losses are infinitesimal; like a building contractor being concerned with a few grains of sand he loses from his fully loaded trucks going down a highway"

"If the grain got in your eye, you'd be concerned." Bill allowed.

"That's a great simile. The sensitive eye being analogous to a sensitive assay," laughed Dr. Kulp. "We'll get it published, but not in the journal to which we first sent it. Some of the reviewers' criticisms were helpful and I believe our revised manuscript is somewhat better than the original.

"The function reviewers and editors should serve is to be certain a manuscript is understandable. It shouldn't be their job to prevent publication of a clear set of experiments. If an author does poor experiments or draws wrong conclusions, it ought not be the reviewers' job to save the author's scientific reputation. A poor paper can tell you something about its author.

"Unfortunately, my views on this subject carry little weight. The Englishmen I met in Bethesda seemed intelligent. I hope a British Journal will prove more intelligent than our journals so far. Let's send it to the British Journal when it is correct and free of typographical errors."

What Jim did not mention to Donna or Bill was the fact that their future job security was in jeopardy until some publications came from their work. His grant-renewal time was approaching and lack of publication could weigh heavily against the award. Unless he could find other sources of money, no grant meant no salaries. His own promotion and a large part of his salary would be dependent upon a regular flow of publications and, as yet, none had materialized.

WINTER

An occasional snowflake floated downward as Bill hurried toward the hospital hoping to be on time. Dr. Fraser's surgical conferences began promptly. Held every Friday morning at seven, the conference kept Dr. Fraser, Chief of Surgery, abreast of the surgical procedures scheduled for the coming week.

Students, house staff, the attending doctors responsible for the patient, as well as certain interested spectators, crowded the small conference room to hear Dr. Fraser's opinion of his house staff's recommendations. The early hour was chosen to interfere as little as possible with the schedule of operations for the day.

As time was short and cases were many, the presentations were brief and informal. Questions could come from anyone in the audience, and, occasionally, a scheduled procedure was put off or altered based upon the discussion which took place. This was the mechanism through which Dr. Fraser could bless or condemn the procedures to be performed by his Surgical Department.

Bill had had to drag himself from bed to attend this conference and he felt lucky to arrive so soon before the conference started and still slip into an empty seat without drawing the attention of the house staff many of whom enjoyed harassing the medical students. He strained to stay awake and follow the discussions as case after case was reviewed in rapid fashion. He concentrated particularly hard when his patients were involved because Dr. Fraser would often ask questions of the medical student assigned to a case.

One of the cases he was to have assisted in operating upon the following Monday was postponed because the attending physician did not feel enough preparative diagnostic data had been obtained. Dr. Fraser quietly reprimanded the house staff involved, pointing out the added costs to the patient the delay would entail.

As all of his cases were discussed early in the conference, he allowed his mind to wander feeling safe from Dr. Fraser's questioning. He thought of Marian and his face flushed with embarrassment thinking how he managed to alienate her just when things seemed to be progressing nicely. Suddenly the part of his mind attending to the conference awakened. Dr. Barry Ward was describing a case operated upon earlier in the week.

"We closed the abdomen after sampling the tumor for pathology. Metastatic lesions were widespread and definitely involved the liver. Surgical pathology has diagnosed the case as an Islet cell carcinoma and that is consistent with the patient's symptoms," Barry told the group.

Bill's attention was caught by the diagnosis. Islet cell carcinoma is an extremely rare form of cancer. Islet cells produce and release Insulin. Tumors of these cells can produce and release excessive amounts of Insulin and such patients develop the symptoms of low blood sugar and the convulsive seizures associated with insulin overdose. In view of the work Bill was doing with Dr. Kulp this patient could be extremely valuable to them. Bill was now fascinated and fully alert.

Barry went on, "The patient, Teddy Runquist, is only sixteen years old. He is already showing signs of jaundice and fluid forming in his abdomen. I don't think he'll last two weeks. It is a damn shame we have nothing to offer this patient."

"But you do!" Bill blurted out.

Though these conferences were informal, it was unusual to have medical students contradicting house staff. A silence followed and all eyes turned toward Dr. Fraser.

"What do you have in mind?" the Chief of Surgery asked the third-year medical student.

"Alloxan," Bill answered. "It could well destroy the islet cells just as it does in our experimental animals. We use it all the time for that in Dr. Kulp's lab."

"I think that has already been tried in man," Dr. Fraser observed with a hint of impatience.

"It has, sir," Barry added, "and it doesn't work."

"You mean Peabody's work?" Bill asked.

Barry nodded.

"He used it all wrong," Bill announced.

"How so?" Dr. Fraser questioned.

"Alloxan is rapidly destroyed in the body," Bill answered." Once destroyed it can't effect islet cells. You have to give large doses rapidly. Peabody gave it to his patients in a slow intravenous drip. It won't work that way."

"Why would he do that?" Dr. Fraser asked.

"I don't know for certain, but I suspect they were being cautious and at that time did not realize how rapidly it was being destroyed in the body." Bill speculated. "The fact that it did not work is all that ever gets reported in the clinical reviews," he added.

"Unfortunately, we don't have the time to discuss this further," Dr. Fraser interrupted. "Barry, get together with this student after conference and get Dr. Kulp and let's see if there is merit to the suggestion."

Bill's heart pounded in his chest and he was suddenly self-conscious as he realized how brash he must appear. Still no one had or reasonably could have taken serious exception to what he had said. He read of alloxan in the scientific literature in preparation for his work with Dr. Kulp. There was nothing else to offer this patient and his suggestion was at least a chance no matter how slim. After all, he was studying to be a doctor and a doctor's primary goal is to help patients. His uneasiness subsided and was gradually replaced by a tinge of self-satisfaction. He was actually getting to contribute to the possible benefit of an ailing human.

The following Monday, Audrey Grovesner Greene sat in her laboratory in Surgical Pathology peering into her microscope. A very impressive instrument it was not merely able to enlarge the image of the tissues under its objectives; but capable of viewing them under all sorts of light directed from all sorts of angles and, in addition, recording what she saw in color or black and white. Large in size, it seemed even larger when Audrey was using it because she was small. Her neat gray hair was knotted in a bun at the back of her head and her frame definitely spare. In keeping with her taut appearance was her no-nonsense manner, piercing gray eyes, and a propensity to pin pomposity to the wall like an insect specimen to a collector's frame. She was Chief of the Surgical Pathology Section of the Department of Surgery. Dr. Thomas Fraser and she had been medical students together in the distant past when few women went into medicine and even fewer into surgery. She had embarked on a career as a surgeon, but gave in to the overwhelming male chauvinism that characterized the field at the time of her early training. Instead, she married a surgeon and developed a career in surgical pathology between babies. She was more famous nationally than any surgeon at Wilder, largely owing to her classic studies of secretory cell tumors. Dr. Fraser was in her laboratory. She lifted her head, hopped off the lab stool and gestured Dr. Fraser toward her microscope.

"See that blue-staining ribbon of cells," she said. "That's characteristic of islet cell cancer. There's not much doubt what we're dealing with, Tom."

Dr. Fraser spoke as he peered into the microscope. "The clinical picture is one of extremely low blood sugars, but it is clouded with a previous history of chronic liver disease following hepatitis. What do you know about alloxan?" he asked.

"Peabody tried it. It doesn't work."

"We have a medical student who challenges that statement."

"On what grounds?"

"Says it was incorrectly used."

"How would he know?" Audrey asked with a hint of annoyance in her voice.

Dr. Fraser looked amused. "He works for Jim Kulp. They use it all the time in their animal research," he said.

Audrey was thoughtful. "Kulp's a careful researcher. Does he concur?"

"Haven't talked with him yet. Wonder if you would mind doing it for me and keeping an eye on this case. This is your field, Aud."

Audrey nodded. "I'll be happy to. Who is the student?"

Dr. Fraser rose from the stool and consulted a small notebook he took from the pocket of his long white coat. "William Michaelson."

"I remember him from the second-year surgery course. He always came into dog surgery looking sick, but he'd make a miraculous recovery by the end of the afternoon. At first I thought he was hung over, but he never smelled of booze. I could not diagnose his problem. Decided he must be squeamish about the using of dogs."

"If that's so, he must be a glutton for punishment working as Kulp's assistant," Dr. Fraser observed. "I'll ask him to come see you. Barry Ward is the resident on that case. Would you like to see them together?"

Audrey was again peering into her microscope. Without looking up she answered, "No. I'll see Michaelson first and if it seems worth pursuing, I'll call the group together."

Late that same afternoon Dr. Greene sat peering into her microscope while Bill Michaelson stared uneasily at her back. When he entered her laboratory, she glanced around briefly and had since been questioning him and simultaneously viewing slides under her microscope. Bill, who found doing more than one thing at a time difficult, was annoyed; he thought her behavior rude.

"Peabody tried it more than once and it failed. What makes you think it is worth trying again?" Audrey asked changing the slide under her microscope.

Bill sneered sarcastically, "Peabody couldn't have screwed it up better if he wanted to fail."

Audrey lifted her head, put on her horn-rimmed glasses and stared at Bill. Pleased to have her undivided attention, he stared back without expression.

"I know Bob Peabody. He's no fool," she said evenly.

"Anyone can make mistakes," Bill shrugged.

"You referring to your judgment of Peabody's alloxan treatment?" Audrey asked.

Realizing Dr. Greene might have misinterpreted his previous statement, Bill answered, "Hell no!"

"Mr. Michaelson," Audrey sounded exasperated, "you needn't try to impress me with profanity. A calm enumeration of the facts will do."

Bill was now embarrassed. Dr. Greene was not one of his favorites. He had felt she was pedantic and excessively self-assured when she had taught him in second year Surgery, but he did realize that her course was well organized and that she seemed genuine in her desire to impart knowledge to her students.

"Dr. Greene," he began, "the fact is alloxan is rapidly destroyed in the bloodstream. Its toxicity to the islet cells is rapidly inactivated. It is also somewhat damaging to other body cells." Momentarily he paused self-consciously realizing Dr. Greene was now intently attending to his every word. "In fact its action on islet cells was discovered when it was being studied for kidney toxicity. In animals you get the most islet cell damage and the least other damage when you give it intravenously and rapidly at the right dosage. Giving it, like Peabody did, in a dilute solution at a slow rate, would favor damage to tissues other than islet cells. I cannot imagine why he chose to administer it that way unless he was ignorant of what I have just told you."

"Perhaps that information was not available to him at the time." Audrey quietly suggested.

"Perhaps, but it is available to us," Bill countered. "That is why I think we ought to try it and do it right."

"How would you propose giving the alloxan?"

"Just as I give it to mice; a rapid intravenous injection."

"I see." Audrey answered and stared at Bill. She thought what an excellent salesman he would make. Despite his obvious annoyance with me his enthusiasm shines through. "Mr. Michaelson," she said, "I'll explore this further. If we decide to do it, I will get in touch with you. Thank you for coming."

She removed her eyeglasses and returned to her microscope.

Interview over, he thought. Don't call us, we'll call you.

The hardly touched evening meal lay jelling in its tray as Teddy Runquist lay stretched out on top of his bed in his faded pajamas and robe. He ached all over. With help from the nurse and attendant, he had tried to walk around the ward, but he just felt too weak and uncomfortable. Why didn't he get well enough to leave this place, he thought. Leave, that was a joke. Where would he go? His father had disappeared and his mother was mostly drunk now. He had no brothers or sisters, and since his dad left there did not seem to be anyone who cared what happened to him. The operation, just one week ago, did not seem to have done much for him. No one told him anything. They just kept asking him when his parents were coming in and he didn't know. His arms were like well-used pin cushions and he seemed to be running out of veins for all the injections and blood samples they were constantly taking. Why weren't they making him better? This was the fourth hospital stay he'd had in the last six months. He'd never make up his school work. He'd already fallen a grade behind. He would quit school. He laughed. For practical purposes I have done just that, he thought. He looked up to see a young man approaching his bed. Not another needle stick. Was this an attendant or a male nurse?

"Are you Teddy Runquist?" the young man asked.

"Yeah. I hope you're not after my veins again," Teddy whined.

"Not at the moment, Teddy. I'm Bill Michaelson, a medical student. Just want to ask you some questions." Bill lowered himself into a bedside chair.

"There's just been a new med student assigned to my case. Are you guys changing again so soon?"

"No, I just want to talk with you." Bill was suddenly unsure what to say to this boy. The newly found confidence arising from his chance to contribute so early in his training faded fast faced with the reality of this seriously ill youth. Though barely sixteen, Teddy resembled a mummy. His wrinkled skin was of an olive green tint and he was emaciated. That's not what a teenager is supposed to look like, Bill thought. Then, too, there was a faint but definite smell; that fetid, livery smell.

Bill had hated liver ever since he had been a child and forced to eat it by an overly enthusiastic parent. He had made a connection between that horrible taste and the human organ when he had dissected a cadaver in anatomy. Whenever he had attended a postmortem on man or animal, that smell eventually suffused his nostrils and he could literally taste it. The animal quarters where he often worked for Dr. Kulp had a similar strong pervasive odor. He could feel himself beginning to gag, but his profound sympathy for the ailing youth before him helped subdue the nausea.

"What do you want to talk about?" Teddy asked.

In truth, Bill had wanted to see just whom he would be treating. He had not seriously considered that he would be doing this; and was surprised when Barry Ward had told him that if alloxan was used, Bill would administer it and be on hand to monitor the patient carefully. Neither could Bill imagine that they would not treat Teddy with alloxan once they confirmed what he had told them during that early morning conference.

As his question was going unanswered, Teddy went on. "They've asked me every question in the books at least three times, but no one answers mine. When am I going to get out of here?"

Bill was horrified. Here he was, talking to Teddy Runquist, yet he had no idea what Teddy had been told about his own condition. This was a living human before him, not a sheaf of papers stuffed into a folder with a number on it. How would he, Bill, feel if they were to exchange places?

"I don't know, Teddy. What have you been told about your sickness?"

"Just that I have a rare disease. I get lots of attention when the doctors come around in groups. I used to anyhow. This past week following the operation, they seem to skip over me. At first I thought it was because I was cured and no longer interesting. Now I'm not sure." He looked squarely at Bill. "What do you think?"

Bill's innards ached. His voice about to crack with emotion, he managed to stammer, "Gee, Teddy, I'm here to learn about your case myself. I'm sort of consulting. I do research, and Dr. Ward wanted me to see you as some of my research might apply to your case. I may have a form of treatment for you."

Teddy sensed that Bill, too, was not going to answer his questions and he lost interest in conversation. He lay back on his pillow and closed his eyes.

Bill was annoyed with himself and, at the same time, relieved. He quietly rose from the chair by Teddy's bed and left. He vowed he would never again make the mistake of approaching a patient without more information concerning what the patient knew of his own case. He would try to make it up to Teddy on his next visit. His self-centered excitement about contributing to Teddy's treatment subsided, tempered by the reality of Teddy Runquist, the human being; or what there was left of him.

"Essentially, then, you confirm all that Mr. Michaelson has told us." Dr. Greene said as she faced Jim Kulp in his office. She thought for a few seconds and then added, "We have absolutely nothing else to offer this patient. I'd be for going ahead. For some odd reason, though, I have the feeling there is sentiment against this. But, then, that's not your problem. Will you help us should we proceed?"

"What do you want from me, exactly?" Jim asked.

"For one thing, we'll need Mr. Michaelson full-time. I understand he helps you in the laboratory."

"That's no problem, Audrey. What else?"

"You'll supervise him? Make sure what he does is reasonable?"

Jim was thoughtful. "Can you spare a technician? We'll need someone to follow the patient's blood sugar levels around the clock. We can teach her the methods but they take time to run and we should monitor them to see if the alloxan is doing anything. Also, if the levels of sugar in the bloodstream fall excessively we'll need to administer some glucose to prevent a hypoglycemic reaction."

"What do you mean?"

"Well, in our animals when we give alloxan and damage islet cells, insulin leeches into the blood stream and occasionally we lose one with low sugar convulsions. A glucose infusion could prevent that."

"Yes, I'll get you a technician." she assured him. "We'll need that kind of data in any case as evidence for alloxan action. That will pacify our critics."

"Who's against this?" Jim asked.

"I'm not sure. Just some rumbling I heard in staff meeting. It seems John Block in Medicine was critical of some surgery of an experimental nature that wasn't too successful last year. He voiced those feelings to Dick Shane. Shane thinks this use of alloxan is more medical than surgical, and suggested we ought to get Medicine to handle it."

"Why don't you? It would get you off the hook."

"Let me remind you, Dr. Kulp, that secretory cell tumors are my domain. Surgery is quite capable of handling this case. We don't need John Block to get us off any non-existent hook."

"I only meant if he was going to be critical, why not let him take the chances."

"It is Shane's fears that have been voiced. I don't know what John thinks."

"Won't this have to come before the Human Research Committee?" Jim asked.

"Damn! Is that committee already operating? I'd heard noises about starting one. Is it a reality this soon?"

"I think it may be, Audrey." Jim laughed. "Yours will probably be the first case to come before it. Aren't you lucky!"

"Lord," she said without smiling, "you do have a warped sense of humor. How much will we need to submit to get this through?"

"I don't know. It's newly formed and I'm not sure what has been decided."

"What prompted its formulation?"

"Grants, Audrey, money from the government. There have been problems which led all federal grants to require a disclaimer. No governmental funds for research unless the human research is done under guidelines set by the government. All schools are gearing up to follow the guidelines. They can't risk losing the research support."

"Who's on the committee?"

"I'll look into it for you."

"I'd certainly appreciate that. If we're going to do this," Audrey added, "we had better move fast. From what Barry Ward reported of his abdominal exploration, we don't have too much time."

"We're not bedeviling this patient, are we?" Jim asked.

"Do you think your treatment has any chance of working?"

Jim thought for several seconds. "A very small chance. Alloxan seems to have a particular toxicity for islet cells. If that's true of cancerous islet cells as well, then it might work."

"Under the circumstances, I believe we'd be remiss not to go ahead. I would if he were my son. You see that this boy gets the best chance for success from this chemical. If others used it unwisely, it's our duty to try and show how it should be used. We have to use a human for this experiment. We don't have an animal model and the boy is going to die if we do nothing."

"I agree, Audrey. That speech ought to convince any committee. Please don't forget it."

Dr. Greene rose to go and giving Jim a wry smile said, "I'm not likely to."

Dr. Alfred Crane wanted to be Dean of the Wilder University Medical School. He was tall, thin, gangly with piercing blue eyes and a friendly smile. He had a sense of humor which he did not hesitate to use, and was the antitheses of the incumbent Dean who he was being groomed to replace. If he played his cards right, the chances were good that his desire would be fulfilled. A local boy, which in these provincial environs was extremely important, and he was Dean Mackenzie's choice for his successor. A good physician, he had done interesting research and gone to the same prestigious northern Medical School the present Dean had attended. In short, he had done everything right. In less than one year Dean Mackenzie would step down. Dr. Crane had merely to coast along and avoid serious controversy.

One assignment he had been given troubled him slightly. He had been made chairman of the newly formed Committee on Human Experimentation a position that could lead to some problems. John Block had been openly critical of the Department of Surgery. Tom Fraser, Surgery's chief, had infuriated John by quietly ignoring him, and now through this committee John was attempting to exert some control over Tom. Alfred Crane had worked for John Block and John assumed that Alfred would do his bidding. Alfred could not afford to alienate anyone as powerful as Tom Fraser; neither could he antagonize John Block who was also powerful by virtue of his political skills rather than a position of power. The Islet cell cancer the Surgical Department was considering treating was creating a problem for Alfred. At any moment, Jim Kulp was coming to see him and a decision would eventually have to be made. Alfred wondered how to settle the conflict with the least enmity fallout in his direction. John Block, when he had gotten wind of the case, said it was a medical problem and should be transferred to Medicine and treated there. Tom Fraser insisted it was surgical and no concern to Medicine. Jim Kulp was coming to see him to determine what responsibilities the Committee on Human

Experimentation had in this case and what would be required to proceed.

In the hope of finding a way out of his dilemma, Alfred had reviewed the medical literature on the use of alloxan in treating islet cell tumors and found three publications relating to the subject; all by a Dr. Robert Peabody. On this basis, one could make a case for the therapy not being experimental, since it had already been done and published, and, therefore, not within the Committee's purview. Alfred liked that, but was sure that tack on his part would upset John because the publications concluded the therapy did not work and Surgery was going to alter the technique in some manner. An amusing aspect of the situation was the fact that the actual treatment was to be done by Dr. Kulp from the Pharmacology department along with a medical student. Alfred was not concerned with their feelings as with the possible exception of the Pathology Department, the Basic Sciences at Wilder were not politically powerful. Wasn't there some way in which he could get Medicine and Surgery to cooperate on this case, he wondered? He was thinking thus when his secretary announced Dr. Kulp.

"Come in, Jim," he flashed his broad friendly smile on Dr. Kulp who knew and liked him.

"What do we have to do to get this thing off the ground, Al?" Jim asked. "This patient may not have much time left."

That's a solution, thought Alfred. If he dies, the problem vanishes. His high forehead wrinkled. "As you well know, Jim, this is a new committee, and we're not exactly set up. This will take careful consideration."

"The patient hasn't much time and what we propose, though admittedly a long shot, is at least something in an otherwise hopeless situation," Jim responded.

"But alloxan is potentially toxic. Its use in man has been limited to date to slow infusions. As I understand it you're proposing the rapid injection of relatively large amounts!"

"Exactly!" Jim exclaimed. "That's the safest way to destroy islet cells in animals."

"Animals, Jim, that's just it There is no evidence it will work the same way in man."

Jim could not believe Alfred was serious. "Of course there's no certainty, but what do we have to lose?" he asked in desperation. He was unaware of Alfred's peculiar problem.

"The Committee will convene as quickly as possible."

"When?"

"Tomorrow afternoon, if I can round up the group."

"Al you realize we don't have much time. The better shape the boy is in the greater are the chances for success."

"I realize your problem. I'm not entirely ignorant of what you propose." Alfred sounded annoyed. "But I, too, have problems of a different sort and I can't just railroad this thing through."

Jim was again struck by the absurdity of what he was hearing. They were dealing with a patient's life and Alfred Crane was concerned with the niceties of committee operation. "Will you call me after your meeting?" he asked.

"Certainly," Alfred answered. Jim was later to wish he had inserted the word "immediately" into the appropriate place in the sentence.

"He's just a kid, Donna, not even seventeen." Bill was standing at the sink washing labware in Dr. Kulp's laboratory. Donna was sitting at her desk calculating results from a past experiment. "He looks as though he were already dead. He's terribly jaundiced, greener than your dress, and he's lost so much weight he's wrinkled. I thought I'd die when he looked me in the eye and asked me to tell him something about his prognosis. His parents are no help. He has no one who gives a damn about him and he senses all is not well."

"How could he feel otherwise?" Donna asked.

"I guess it's a blessing they're keeping him heavily sedated now. He sleeps most the time. I first visited him when he was lucid, much to my discomfort. I just wanted to see the patient we'd be working on. It was a mistake for me to see him like that. I get less upset by sick patients when I have a specific reason to visit them like getting a blood sample or getting the answer to a specific question. Then it's less personal."

"That's probably what they mean about not getting emotionally involved," Donna speculated.

"I suppose. I do wish we'd get on with the treatment if we're going to do it. The suspense is awful."

"When will you know?"

"I don't know. I almost wish I'd never opened my mouth in that Surgical Conference."

"That's nonsense. The whole reason for our being is to develop ideas that will be of use in the clinic; ideas that will help sick people," Donna replied.

"That sounds great, but the reality of taking ideas from animal experiments into man can be difficult. I never considered it carefully before. When I inject these mice with alloxan, about twenty percent die. That's no problem. Mice are cheap and the eighty percent who survive are adequate for our experiments. Now we're talking about one chance in five of my killing Tommy when I inject the stuff. That's frightening."

"Not really. Not when you know the alternative."

"If he dies of his cancer, Donna, I didn't kill him."

"Didn't you? When you withhold a possible cure for Tommy, isn't that worse than nudging him over the brink?"

"Put in those terms, I suppose so." Bill fell silent for a time as he rinsed glassware with distilled water. Finally he sighed. "I suppose. I can honestly say I'd treat someone from my own family the same way. There really isn't a better way to judge the rightness of my behavior." He shook his head. "I hope I won't have too many decisions like this to think about."

"I suspect there will be many more you'll make as a physician," Donna speculated. She then added, "Something has been troubling Andy lately, and I suspect it is of a similar nature. He hasn't confided in you, has he?"

"No, but I don't see a lot of him. An occasional noon lecture together. That's all."

"It's not like Andy to hold out on me," Donna mused. "I wish I knew what his problem is."

"Maybe he's just tired. There's lots of night work on obstetrics. Babies come at all hours they tell me."

Dr. Kulp entered the laboratory. "Bill," he said, "glad you're here. I've been wanting to talk about Tommy Runquist."

"Me too," Bill nodded. "I've been so busy I haven't had the chance to see you since last week. Guess I really started something in that Friday Surgical Conference."

Jim smiled broadly. "You sure as hell did. I'm glad you were there. Otherwise we never would have heard of that case until autopsy."

"What do you think of my suggestion?" Bill asked.

"It's certainly worth a try," Jim answered.

"I didn't expect to get it dumped in my lap when I suggested it," Bill admitted.

"No one over there has ever used alloxan," Jim pointed out. "They needed your expertise."

Bill could not tell whether Dr. Kulp was making fun of him; but, as he saw no sign of a smile on the doctor's face, he assumed he was serious. "I don't feel like an expert," he said.

"Bill," Jim confided, "you'll soon realize that there is so much in medicine that most clinician's knowledge of any subject is apt to be superficial. Expertise is relative, and direct experience is the best teacher if you are observant and receptive. You rightly pointed out to them that the previous human studies completely neglected inactivation rates. Therefore, you are an expert. It doesn't mean you know very much, just more than they do."

"Do they plan to treat him with alloxan?" Donna asked.

"I just met with Al Crane," Jim answered. "He told me the Human Research Committee will meet to discuss it tomorrow."

"And then we get a decision?" Bill asked.

"I sure hope so," Jim answered. "I hear Tommy is sinking. The tumor must be choking off blood supply to vital organs. What kind of a dose do you think we should administer?"

"The same as I give the mice." Bill answered. "That's fifty milligrams per kilo."

"That's about two and one half grams," Jim figured," assuming Teddy's fifty kilograms. Let's give forty. That would be two grams."

"Why do you want to decrease it?" Bill asked.

"Because they made me responsible and I'm naturally cautious," Jim answered with a grin.

"What are you afraid of?" Bill asked.

"I honestly don't know. Just cautious. Species vary in their sensitivity to drugs. Forty seems like a lot to me especially if you bang it in fast and you should. Don't you agree, Bill."

"Yes sir, I sure do." Bill answered with a grin.

The Human Research Committee was comprised of a representative from each of the five major clinical departments. Alfred Crane could not convene the group until Thursday afternoon.

Dr. John Block, representing Medicine, asked the first question after Alfred Crane opened the meeting and Dr. Audrey Grovesner Greene, representing Surgery, presented Tommy Runquist's plight and the proposed course of action.

"Who will administer the alloxan and who will be following the patient?" he asked.

Audrey answered. "Dr. James Kulp of Pharmacology who uses the drug in his research work has agreed to help us."

"Don't you think this would be better done under the auspices of Medicine? After all, Audrey, it's a medical problem," John announced.

"How so, John?" Audrey asked.

"You are treating the condition with a drug, not a surgical procedure," John replied.

"That's nonsense," Audrey countered. "This patient has had several surgical procedures over the past months and is admittedly beyond surgical help for his primary problem at least. We're recommending a last-ditch attempt to stave off what may well be inevitable. We're not terribly optimistic, but we feel this is an opportunity to use alloxan properly, and we hope to destroy cancer cells with it. If we succeed the condition may again be operable. Besides the only work published in this field is by a Surgeon."

"You just said it wasn't done properly," said John with a smirk.

"Dr. Block," she replied, "I do not intend arguing with you about the relative merits of medicine and surgery as a form of therapy. That is a useless exercise." Audrey hesitated a moment and then asked, "why do you want this case?"

John Block had no intention of answering the question honestly. With all the new governmental guidelines for research, he saw opportunities for money pouring out of Washington. Through contacts in the nation's capital, he had been aware of a trend toward the financial support of clinical studies. He saw this as a vehicle for building up the Medical School which he envisioned the Department of Medicine would control. With Alfred Crane, the new Dean in his pocket, he could take over as the Chief of Medicine. The present Chief would undoubtedly soon resign as he was in poor health.

"It's obvious to me it's a medical problem," he answered smugly.

"Well, it is not obvious to me, John," Audrey replied and flashed one of her rare and charming smiles at him.

"In view of the age of the patient," said Gerald Porter who represented Pediatrics," one could call this a pediatric problem, but we sure as hell don't want it, Audrey."

"Thank you, Jerry," she answered. "What do we need to get going with this project?"

"We'll need to see your protocol," John Block said, "and we, as a committee, will have to pass on it. Isn't that so, Al?" he asked as an afterthought realizing he was usurping the chairman's prerogative.

"Quite so, John. Audrey, if you will supply all the members of the Committee with your protocol, we'll review it, and we can go on from there."

Audrey frowned. "May I suggest that to save time, which is running out on Tommy Runquist, that we have Jim Kulp meet with us and dispense with the formal protocol for now."

"We'll need a written record for the committee," John insisted.

"You will have it, John," Audrey replied impatiently. "But is it necessary before we start treatment? If we agree in principle, we can take care of the details later. As a matter of fact, in the interest of time, I would like to get Jim Kulp to speak with us right now." She rose from the table.

"That's not really necessary," Alfred Crane asserted with a pained look. "If the patient's that badly off, aren't you doomed to failure anyway? You may be doing the therapy a disservice using it on so sick a patient. Why not wait for a better subject?"

"Islet cell carcinomas are scarcer than hen's teeth," Audrey replied in disbelief. "I do not see why this Committee cannot respond rapidly when there is a demonstrated need as there is now. If there is a real difference between surgeons and medical men, it may well be in the inordinate amount of time you 'pill-pushers' spend trying to decide what to do. We know Tommy is not going to get any better. Please, let us come to a quick decision." She pointedly addressed her plea to Al and John.

"I agree with Audrey. Let's move." Jake Bourne said with impatience. "Let's see Jim Kulp if the rest of this group needs him to hold their hand while we come to a decision. Personally, I don't need him. I go along with Audrey's proposal right now."

"Thank you Jake," Audrey sighed. "What do we need, Al? A majority?"

"That's one of many things this Committee has to resolve," Alfred answered. "How do we go about ruling on requests? We're obviously not ready yet."

"Then let's improvise," Jake suggested. "There are five voting members of this Committee. If three agree, we go. Audrey and I vote 'yes'. What about you Jerry and John? The shrink's not here."

"Slow down, Jake," Alfred admonished, "we can't do it like that."

"Why the hell not?" Jake retorted. "Just 'cause we move quickly doesn't mean we haven't thought about it. I've sat through this entire meeting without opening my mouth. What do you think I was doing? Daydreaming?"

John, ignoring Jake's sarcasm, asked, "What do you mean by 'five' voting members? We're six."

"Bullshit!" Jake exploded. "You and Al are both from Medicine. One of you can't vote. I assume Al as chairman is purely administrative."

"I'm not so sure about that," John replied.

Despite the attempts to speed things up, progress deteriorated and no definite decision was reached. A time for reviewing a verbal or written protocol was tentatively set for the following afternoon. The group dispersed and Alfred Crane and John Block held a private discussion in John's office.

"I get the distinct impression you're not in favor of Audrey' proposal," said Alfred with a smile.

"The approach is a good one. From what I'm hearing alloxan wasn't used intelligently, and it would be damned interesting to see if it could destroy the islet cell cancer cells. I doubt it will do much for the patient, though. He's too far along. Under Medicine, it could prove a valuable experiment."

"Valuable to whom?" Alfred asked.

John gave him a wary glance. "Al," he said, "you had better recognize some facts if you expect smooth sailing in the next few months." He paused and the two men stared at each other. Alfred looked away. John went on. "With you Dean and me Chief of Medicine and Medicine in control of this School and teaching hospital, we can make this a first-rate medical school. If we let some of these other departments have too much say, we run the chance of becoming just another second-rate southern school."

Alfred Crane bristled inwardly. John Block was a "damn Yankee" who had recently migrated, and Alfred, a born Southerner though educated in the North, did not appreciate John's attitude. Nor did he care for John's reference to a possible lack of smoothness in his ascension to the Deanship, especially since he well recognized the validity of the threat. He would have to cooperate with John at least until he was Dean. After that, he would see.

Following a seemingly endless amount of wrangling, paper shuffling, telephoning, and walking from one part of the University complex to another for brief meetings, Audrey Greene and James Kulp were finally given the institutions permission to treat Tommy Runquist. This had taken till Saturday afternoon and they were then frustrated by still being unable to contact Tommy's mother or father for parental permission. In desperation, they decided themselves to assume the standard operative permission form which had been secured on Tommy's hospital admission would cover their treatment. Tommy had now been unconscious for over twenty-four hours and showed no sign of improvement. Owing to the lateness of the hour, they decided to get an early start next morning. As she had stated she would, Audrey called Bill Michaelson.

On Sunday, the small empty four-bed ward set aside for the procedure and follow up studies, had an eerie quality. Three empty beds were pushed to the side and Tommy lay in the middle of the brightly lit room. As the surgical technician Audrey had promised Jim Kulp was off for the weekend, Donna Beardsley was present to analyze the blood samples for sugar. She had set up all the needed equipment at the bedside to save time and steps. Some pretreatment control blood samples were taken, and shortly after noon they were ready to administer the alloxan. A long needle had been secured in the large femoral vein in Tommy's groin with a saline infusion flowing through it to insure access to Tommy's bloodstream. Bill and Donna were clothed in sterile green operating caps, shirts, pants, masks and gowns to minimize the chances of infecting Tommy.

Bill dissolved the alloxan powder in a beaker of sterile salt solution wearing sterile rubber gloves which made him feel clumsy. He drew the solution into a syringe through a valve which he controlled with a tiny lever. As the capacity of the largest available syringe was far less than the volume of solution to be injected, the plan was to push the plunger with the valve positioned so that the solution entered the vein, turn the valve lever to the proper position, pull the plunger to refill the syringe from the beaker, and repeat this until all the solution had been drawn from the beaker and administered. Donna was holding the tubing below the surface of the solution in the beaker so that no air would enter the syringe. Dr. Kulp was to time the period necessary to force the drug into Tommy's bloodstream. Tension was high.

Bill's hands were shaking as he disconnected the saline infusion and connected the syringe to the femoral needle.

"Don't shake the needle out of the vein," Dr. Kulp admonished.

"Are you ready?" Dr. Greene inquired. She added, "Relax, William, you will do this properly."

No one at Wilder called him "William." That simple act recalled childhood feelings which were calming.

"Start!" Bill nodded toward Dr. Kulp as he forced the first syringe load of solution into Teddy. All went smoothly and sixty-five seconds later the entire volume of solution had been administered.

Earlier, Dr. John Block had won a single concession in the protocol. He had insisted that ascorbic acid be administered intravenously three minutes after the last of the alloxan was given to destroy any that had not been inactivated by then, thereby decreasing its toxicity. Bill was concerned that alloxan's action on the cancer, also, might be impaired and wondered why Dr. Kulp had accepted this concession.

"Block was mistaken," Dr. Kulp informed him with a smile. "If anything, ascorbic acid will increase alloxan's action. I didn't have the heart to correct him."

Three minutes later, the ascorbic acid was administered. Through it all, Tommy lay quietly breathing slowly, oblivious to the activity around him.

For the first half-hour following the alloxan administration a great deal of attention was focused on Tommy. Pulse, blood pressure and respirations were noted at five minute intervals. The eyes of the four observers seldom left their subject. With the exception of a blotchy redness which appeared on Tommy's neck, shoulders and chest for a few moments five minutes after the injections, there was nothing to note. Tension slowly gave way to disappointment as it became apparent nothing dramatic seemed to be happening. The four observers felt this and agreed it was an inappropriate reaction. In laboratory animal experiments nothing would be seen for several hours and then it was the glucose levels in the blood that told the story.

Drs. Greene and Kulp gave telephone numbers where they could be reached and left Bill and Donna the task of obtaining, recording and analyzing data at specified intervals. At first the time passed quickly and soon the small ward became filled with the paraphernalia of the laboratory procedures being conducted—specimen bottles, syringes, needles test tubes and pipettes. As this was a Sunday, there were few visitors to the wards and they were able to conduct their studies without interruption.

For a time, observations were made at fifteen minute intervals and Bill and Donna were kept busy. Later, fewer observations had to be made and the frantic activity gave way to a routine of work and wait. Boredom set in and by twenty-four hours Bill sent Donna home as he was able to handle the work and it was now Monday morning and neither of them had slept. Tommy remained in coma and the only apparent difference was a change in the character of his breathing. His respirations were more rapid and forceful. The expired air was causing his vocal cords to vibrate, and each time he breathed there was a groaning sound. As this had come on very gradually, it did not alarm Bill.

He had managed to secure a degree of privacy by pulling curtains over the windows of the nursing station and keeping the ward door closed. At mid-morning, he decided to try and get some rest and lay on one of the empty beds. He quickly drifted off to sleep. Within a few minutes, he sat bolt upright in response to a very strong stimulus; sudden, absolute silence! Tommy's groans had ceased. He jumped from the bed. He put his hand on Tommy's chest and thought he could feel a heart beat. Panic rose and intelligent thought refused to come. Before he could decide what he should do, Tommy breathed again.

What a great doctor you are, he thought. The incident took less than a minute though it seemed much longer and completely dispelled any drowsiness Bill had felt. The respirations became irregular now. Tommy would breathe for a few minutes steadily and then would stop breathing for half a minute. This irregularity became so regular that it ceased to alarm Bill.

The levels of glucose in the blood had been rising slowly ever since the alloxan had been administered owing to a glucose infusion that had been started to prevent low blood sugar. The twenty-nine hour sample showed a marked fall, a sign they had all hoped for. Bill called Dr. Kulp who came to the ward immediately.

"You sure you didn't slow the glucose infusion?" he asked Bill.

"No, Sir. Also I ran duplicates from the blood sample. Donna's back and she's running a check now," Bill answered excitedly. "I think the stuff is working!" He could hardly stand still.

"Has Tommy shown any change?" Jim Kulp inquired.

"Except for his breathing, no," Bill replied.

Donna had finished her analysis and confirmed Tommy's blood sugar data.

"Great," Jim shouted. "The alloxan is working." He turned to see Dr. Greene entering the room. "It seems to be working. The sugar is falling just as it does at first in our lab animals." He beamed at Audrey.

"Is he in any danger of hypoglycemia?" Audrey asked.

"We have a steady glucose infusion and can speed it up if we need to," Jim assured her.

"How is he?" she asked Bill. She went to the bedside and peered at Tommy. "He looks even more jaundiced to me. Doesn't he look yellower than yesterday?"

"If he is the change has been too gradual for me to see," Bill replied.

"I think you are right," Jim answered soberly. "Just our luck. The drug works, but the patient is too far gone to recover. Why did it take us so damn long to get started?"

"I doubt whether a few days would have made much difference." Audrey pondered. "Tommy was pretty badly off at the time Barry Ward explored his abdomen. Still, had we known of this approach we might have moved faster. Next time we will, though next time will probably be somewhere else with others in attendance. That's why," she added, turning towards Bill, "you must keep good records and publish this. You look terrible. Go home and get some sleep. Donna, Jim and I can manage."

"I would appreciate a chance to shower and change clothes," he admitted, "if you're sure you can spare me."

The warmth of the early afternoon sunshine soothed Bill as he walked towards his room with that wonderful feeling of accomplishment of a job well done. He wasn't sleepy. He was keyed up, wide awake and strangely relaxed all at once. When he luxuriated in a long hot shower, a drowsiness did overtake him, and he slipped naked between the sheets for a short nap. He awoke and was surprised to find that daylight had gone. He'd slept twelve hours. He dressed hurriedly and ran to the hospital through deserted streets.

He was surprised to find the four-bed ward dark and dismayed to find it empty when he located and turned on the lights. All vestiges of the work they had done were gone. Had he come to the wrong floor? He checked in the nursing station, but the strange night nurse did not know the whereabouts of his patient. A nursing supervisor appeared and on questioning, simply announced that Tommy Runquist had expired. Why didn't they call me, he wondered?

Confused and depressed, he left the ward. He walked along a hospital corridor wondering what to do next when he heard noises coming from one of the doctor's offices he was passing. The sound which caught his attention was a moaning sobbing sound.

"No, I won't have you cutting my baby, my Tommy," a slurred voice cried.

He heard Barry Ward's voice reply, "But, Mrs. Runquist, it might be very important to future cases. Tommy would not have died for nothing. Please let us do an autopsy?"

"No cutting! My baby's dead. Tommy's gone. Will cutting bring him back? No," she said with finality.

Bill had heard enough. He ran to the Pharmacology Department where he unceremoniously burst into Dr. Kulp's office to find Jim and Dr. Greene conversing. "Why didn't you call me?" he demanded.

Audrey Greene turned toward him with a patient but frosty stare. "What could you have done that was more important than catching up on your sleep? You are still required to fulfill the duties of your third-year surgical clerkship."

Somewhat chastened, Bill asked in a calmer tone, "What happened?"

"The inevitable," she answered. "He just stopped breathing. None of us felt heroic efforts to save him were in order. That child's suffering is over."

"We can't locate his father and his mother is against an autopsy," Jim added. "Barry is trying, but if we don't get an autopsy, the fall in blood sugar isn't enough evidence for alloxan action by itself. His death and our work may add up to nothing."

"I don't believe Barry is making any progress from what I overheard just now," Bill told them. He and Jim Kulp looked dejected.

Audrey glared at the men. "When I was a resident," she said, "if needs be, we were known to steal a Post."

"How'd you get away with that?" Bill asked.

"We stole tissue through the rectum or vagina if female," she answered. "It wasn't easy or ideal, but it was done. Tommy's incision from the exploration never healed well. It would be easy to get tissue through that."

"Let's do it," Bill pleaded excitedly. "We really must find out what we did to that cancer?"

"And the normal tissue," Jim added.

"You don't need to convince me," Audrey smiled. "I'm as curious as you. We can't hurt Tommy any more, and I would like to give some meaning to all that child has been through. His idiot parents hardly deserve consideration, but for God's sake be discreet. They're just the ones to sue."

Barry Ward joined them and the four proceeded to the morgue. They located the shriveled body in the refrigerated storage, and the men lifted Tommy's remains and placed them on the gleaming stainless steel autopsy table. They had spoken to George, the autopsy room diener, and obtained the keys they needed for their work. George was delighted that this was not to be a postmortem but just a "viewing of the body" that did not require his services. George had been at Wilder almost as long as Audrey. They were longtime acquaintances, so there had been no problems thus far.

"This wound has practically disrupted," noted Barry, cutting the remaining stitches with a scissors. He and Audrey were gloved and took turns reaching through the incision and feeling for the various organs they desired to sample. Audrey did not have a long reach and there were moments when her arm was inside Tommy's body up to her shoulder. Her pink cheek against Tommy's olive colored belly produced a startling contrast. At such times Audrey would close her eyes and describe the organs she was feeling for the benefit of those present and a wire recorder. Within a half hour, samples of most of the organs they desired were obtained.

"Can you feel much of the original tumor mass?" Jim asked Barry.

"It's hard to tell." Barry answered. "It was so diffuse in the first place that it would be impossible to say there was a difference from what we saw at exploration. I hope we can tell something from the microscopic appearance of the tissue sections.

They closed the wound with some new stitches and hoped no one would look too closely to determine just when the stitches had been placed. With the tissue samples safely covered with formalin fixative and the body again reposing in the cold atmosphere of the refrigerator, they left the morgue feeling they had made the best of a bad situation. Had permission for a postmortem examination been granted, they could have opened the abdomen and viewed its contents and been better able to sample the tumor mass. It is even possible Barry might have been able to see a change in the appearance of the tumor. As it was they could not even be sure the samples they had taken surreptitiously were tumor. Only later microscopic examinations might reveal how successful their treatment and this wee small hour of the morning mission to the morgue had been. In the past, Bill had heard Dr. Kulp express himself on the many difficulties involved in doing medical research on human patients. He was beginning to understand.

Terry Brown managed to squeak past Biochemistry. Not proud of his grade, he was thankful that hurdle was behind him. This winter session Terry faced pathology and pharmacology. He liked the subject matter far better than biochemistry and was determined to heed the Dean's advice to work hard from the onset.

The courses had been in session only two weeks and already he felt behind. There was so much material to learn. If he were studying the list of drugs which cause blood vessels to constrict and sorting them out as to their effects on other organs, how they are administered, their effects on other drugs, he should have been studying the conditions which cause high blood pressure, and what diseased vessels look like when cut, stained and viewed under the microscope. This was fascinating material; but, between the two courses, there was just too damn much of it. Others have done it before me, he thought. I'll survive somehow.

At one o'clock, he sat in a lecture room listening to Dr. Anthony Lewis expound on autonomic drugs. He tried to stay alert because he was to use some of these drugs this afternoon in the Pharmacology laboratory. They were going to observe changes in the dog's blood pressure in response to the drugs they would administer.

The class was divided into small laboratory groups and each member of the group had a turn to prepare the animal. Today was Terry's turn. He would have to cut down on an artery and tie a cannula, a rigid tube, in the vessel so that the animals blood was in direct contact with a salt solution within a small flexible hose. The plastic hose, several feet in length, was connected to a vertical glass "U" tube partially filled with mercury. The mass of the mercury was such that it counterbalanced the dog's blood pressure. On the side of the "U" tube away from where the salt solution was in contact with the mercury, a float with a rigid wire sat atop the mercury. With fluctuations in the dog's blood pressure the wire bobbed up and down. A celluloid tip attached to the wire recorded these changes by rubbing continuously against a moving soot-coated paper surface. The smoked paper was mounted on a drum which was rotated by a clock-like mechanism called a kymograph. Currently, more convenient and expensive electrical recording devices are used, but the lessons learned are much the same.

Terry, had never before been designated as "surgeon" and he was unsure how he would perform. He imagined himself decked out in the green scrub suit issuing orders to a group of less skilled surgical assistants and sexy operating room nurses. His mind was thus occupied when he heard his name called and noticed the eyes of his fellow students turned toward him in amusement.

"Mr. Brown, please answer that question?" Dr. Lewis had the habit of interrupting his lecture to ask questions, especially if he thought his students were not paying attention. The lecture hour just after lunch provided a challenge to any lecturer to keep his audience awake. Tony Lewis was a kindly man and did not enjoy embarrassing students. He noted Terry's confusion and suspected he had not heard the question.

"Mr. Brown," he asked," how much one-one hundredth percent solution of epinephrine would you give your dog to give five micrograms of epinephrine?"

Terry heard the question but did not answer.

"Well?" Dr. Lewis persisted.

"I can't do that calculation," Terry admitted.

"Sure you can," Dr. Lewis coaxed. "Come up here to the black board."

Terry rose and went forward shaking his head. When he reached the chalk board, Dr. Lewis handed him a piece of chalk. Terry stood motionless, his back to the class.

"What is the concentration of epinephrine in a one-one hundredth percent solution?" Dr. Lewis asked.

"I don't know," Terry answered.

"All right," Dr. Lewis said, "let's start at the beginning. A one hundred percent solution contains one hundred grams per one hundred milliliters. Using that reference point," Tony wrote it on the board, "how much epinephrine would be in a one percent solution?"

"I don't know," Terry answered.

Dr. Lewis's mouth fell open. "Come on," he asked, "do you mean to tell me if I borrowed two hundred dollars from you at two percent interest annually you couldn't calculate what I owed you at the end of the year?"

"Oh sure," Terry answered, "two percent of two hundred, that's the same as one percent of one hundred."

Dr. Lewis froze. He shook his head. This was a medical student: a college graduate! A student in one of the back rows raised his hand. Dr. Lewis nodded.

"Where do you learn to do problems like this?" he asked.

Without sarcasm Dr. Lewis answered, "You start in kindergarten and work your way up."

"But what if you didn't learn it? Where can you go now?" the student persisted.

"I guess you have to find an elementary mathematics book," Dr. Lewis answered. "I can't remember which grade taught percentage problems." He continued to stare at the class. Finally he asked, "How many of you can't do that problem?"

Slowly hands began to appear. In a class of seventy students ten had already raised their hands. Dr. Lewis stood shaking his head. One of the delinquent students must have become annoyed with the doctor's apparent disbelief.

"Why do we have to know this stuff anyway?" he asked.

"How do you intend to give your patients the proper amount of a drug?" Dr. Lewis replied.

"The dose is usually written on the bottle," the student answered.

"Not always," Dr. Lewis countered. "What if it isn't?"

"I'll ask a nurse," came the answer.

Dr. Lewis stood looking at the class. There were no smiles. He did not think they were joking with him; yet he could not believe they were serious. He was trying to think of the proper thing to say when a buzzer signaled the end of the hour.

"Class dismissed," he said with a sigh.

During the interval between his lecture and the laboratory exercise, Dr. Lewis reported the episode to the other pharmacology faculty members. Jim Kulp and Rodney Barret did not seem surprised, but Bob Mettlar refused to believe it. He was sure the students were joking. Bob's attitude made Tony Lewis begin to wonder if, indeed, they had been fooling him.

"We'll have a chance to see how they calculate doses in the dog experiment coming right up," Jim Kulp observed as they all started toward the student laboratory.

The student laboratory exercises were conducted in two large rooms at the end of the corridor. The laboratories were divided into student work stations and each station had its own dog board and smoked paper kymograph. To save time the staff had anesthetized the dogs and secured them to the dog boards with ties. The animals were under deep anesthesia and would never again awaken. They had been obtained from dog pounds where they had been scheduled for extermination.

Terry Brown's group was supervised by Jim Kulp. He was pleased to see Terry go right to work in a manner that suggested he had prepared and knew what he was doing. Terry dissected out the carotid artery in the dog's neck and had it cannulated and connected to the mercury manometer before any other group.

Dr. Lewis's story of Terry's mathematical deficiency had not surprised Jim as he had noted that with few exceptions, doctors did not seem to be mathematically oriented. He decided he would watch carefully as they administered their first injection of epinephrine to the dog. A miscalculation might produce some peculiar results and make the students realize the importance of being able to calculate dosages properly.

When Terry's group was ready to administer their first dose, it was clear they were far ahead of the other groups and were clearly pleased. There was lighthearted bantering between Terry and the "surgeons" in surrounding groups concerning their dogs dying of old age before the surgery was completed.

As Jim predicted, Terry's group erroneously calculated the dose for the first injection. They used a ten times too concentrated solution and gave ten times too much volume. Thus, they administered one hundred times the amount of epinephrine called for in the experimental protocol. Jim felt certain the excessive dose would not kill the animal but would demonstrate a maximal response that was clearly greater than the other groups would see. He could then point out their mistake and chastise them for an error which with another drug might prove fatal. Even Jim was not prepared for what followed.

Terry's dog was a very large one. It had a large and powerful heart and the massive dose of epinephrine produced an amazing increase in the force of contraction which increased the dog's blood pressure until it exceeded the inertia of all the mercury in the "U" tube manometer. The students and Dr. Kulp stood fixed; fascinated, as the float and wire marker popped out of the "U" tube followed by a fountain of clear salt solution which quickly turned crimson as arterial blood sprayed the environs. Terry, seeing his triumphant surgical efforts coming to naught, sprang into action. He grasped the open end of the "U" tube and planted his thumb firmly on top. This stopped the flow.

"Midge," he shouted to his student assistant, "put a clamp back on the artery!"

Midge, who had been watching with hypnotic fascination, came out of her trance and complied. Within seconds, the dog's exsanguination had been averted.

The mess took time to rectify and Terry's group slipped from the furthest ahead to the furthest behind. Jim watched as the subdued students cleaned up and proceeded with the experiment. He noted how carefully they checked and double checked amongst themselves the doses to be given, and would even occasionally consult with him. How could anyone doubt the value of student laboratories after seeing the lesson learned this afternoon, he wondered. No book could teach such a lesson. He would never forget that crimson fountain.

"Terry," Jim said when the group had finally finished the experiment, "you and your group handled that emergency well. I am proud of you for that part. Find anyone in your class who needs help in the mathematics of dosage calculation, and we'll schedule some extra classes to be certain you can do them before the mid-term examination. One or two sessions should do it. It isn't difficult. I promise you some dosage questions on the mid-term.

"Yes, sir, and thanks," Terry said with a sanguine grin; arterial dog blood had dried on his cheek.

A puzzled John Block placed the medical journal he had been reading on the desk in front of him, removed his glasses and leaned back in his chair. Nearly midnight, he alone manned the Department of Medicine. He was not on duty. He simply worked long hours and tonight he was reading the current journals to be certain he was abreast of anything new in the field of kidney research. What puzzled him was that no researcher, as yet, had been able to produce an animal model of headache remedy kidney damage, known as analgesic nephrotoxicity to the medical profession.

In certain areas of the world, including the southeastern United States, all too many inhabitants suffer from this condition. It is caused by the routine excessive intake of certain headache remedies. This seemingly innocuous habit can grow to such proportions that the end result is a loss of kidney function and death or the necessity for lifelong dialysis treatments.

Afflicted patients usually tell of ingesting ten to twenty daily doses for as many years. Often they work in noisy, stress producing occupations such as assembly lines or they may do piecework in a garment factory. Occasionally, as in the case of Marie Barrett, the stresses of home and hearth are sufficient. At first, the medication is taken to combat headaches and minor physical discomforts, but soon they are taken prophylactically to prevent symptoms and promote well being. As most of the ingredients of these concoctions are excreted from the body by way of the kidney, that organ has to deal with very large quantities over a very long time. All too frequently this organ is asked to exceed its excretory capacity and is destroyed.

This condition was gaining wide recognition and the kidney literature contained many studies, but no one was certain just which substance in these preparations was responsible for the kidney damage. One group, with whom John sided, blamed phenacetin. Others pointed out that since these preparations contained aspirin as well, it was not realistic to blame phenacetin without more specific data. As is too often in the case of scientific debate, sides were drawn, polemics proliferated and more heat than light was generated.

Though no one as yet had produced the kidney damage experimentally, John knew phenacetin had to be the culprit. Why shouldn't he be the first? If he were to give rats large doses of phenacetin over a prolonged period and they were to develop kidney lesions similar to those found in man at autopsy, wouldn't that settle the question? He would get credit for being the first investigator to do so and his already lofty national image would soar even higher. He sighed aloud and a warmth suffused his body.

He would enlist the aid of Harry Tatum, professor of pathology, to do the pathological evaluations. Harry would jump at a chance to collaborate with him and would pose no threat to his position as senior author. Everyone would know it was his work and that Harry was merely a flunky engaged to do the routine pathology.

John thought, we'll give a large dose of phenacetin daily to rats by stomach tube for a ten week period. Then we'll kill the rats and have Harry study their kidneys for signs of damage. John slowly became aware of sounds coming from Peter Markley's office next door. He rose, walked out into the hall, and looked in to see Peter.

"You're here late." John said.

"You startled me," Peter gasped. "I didn't know anyone else was around."

"What's up?" John asked.

"An emergency dialysis. A surgical patient had renal shutdown. The schedule is so full we decided to do her tonight. I hope her kidneys open up quickly."

"Peter, have you been following the phenacetin renal toxicity story closely?" John asked.

"I know we have too many patients on dialysis because they abused the analgesic drugs. Why?"

"I don't understand why someone hasn't already done it, but I plan to answer this question once and for all," John announced. He went on to tell Peter of his plan for the rat experiment. He liked to use members of his staff as sounding boards. He knew Peter, though not research oriented, was intelligent and would not hesitate to point out any flaws he could see. The two discussed his plan for some time despite the lateness of the hour.

The result was a modified plan far better designed to give information. John would use three groups of rats. To one, he would administer phenacetin. To another he would give aspirin, an ingredient also present in many of the offending preparations. To a third group, he would give acetaminophen, the substance phenacetin was converted to in the body, and which was itself gaining prominence and popularity as a new headache remedy known as Tylenol. He would give equal doses of the three and find out which produced the kidney lesion. Yes, sir, he thought, I like the idea of being the first to produce this lesion in animals.

A few miles away neither Janet nor Jim could get to sleep. Side by side, each conscious of the other's breathing, neither of them knew whether the other lay awake.

Janet finally broke the silence. "Honey, you awake?"

"Yes," Jim replied.

"I've been lying here thinking," Janet said. "What happens when your current grant runs out?"

"That's at least two years off," her husband answered. "Aren't you worrying prematurely?"

"Am I, Jim? You'll have to apply for a renewal early next fall, and if you don't have a manuscript accepted for publication by then, what are your chances of getting it?"

"Not good," he admitted, "but certainly by then I should have something in press."

"You don't sound very convincing."

"I know," he admitted, "I think there's a conspiracy to prevent my publication because it will embarrass the big shots in the field."

"Can't Bob Mettlar help?" Janet asked. "He's well known and influential."

"Not in the micro-insulin assay field," Jim answered with a sigh. "But stop worrying, we'll get published."

"I'm sure you will, but in time for your grant renewal?"

"God I hope so! If I lose the grant, I lose Donna and Bill and a quarter of my salary."

"Won't the school make it up? Your salary, at least?"

"In theory," Jim answered, Wilder is supposed to pay my salary, but if the same thing happens to too many of us at the same time, they couldn't. That's why I'm seriously considering a consulting job offer."

Not far from Wilder University was the city of Chester. In that city of one hundred thousand population was the Rule Pharmaceutical Company which manufactured and sold one product, an APC. The product, a mixture of aspirin, phenacetin and caffeine, had been marketed in the form of a powder for thirty years, ever since Mr. Rule first mixed the powders in his corner drug store to treat the hangovers of his hard-drinking friends. Such powders are popular in the Southeast where they are felt by their users to be superior to the same substances in tablet form. A small Company, Rule had offered Jim a job consulting.

"You're really going to work for them?" Janet asked. "I thought you said you would never work for a drug company?"

Jim was silent a moment before answering. "I did say that, but I was referring to ethical drug companies. They sell prescription drugs. Rule sells only one over-the-counter preparation; an APC powder."

"I don't understand. What's the difference?"

"I said I wouldn't work for the ethical drug industry because for it to survive as a business it must sell people drugs they don't need. Since prescription drugs are highly active and powerful agents, they can do much harm. If drug use were limited to necessary use, ninety percent of the ethical drug companies would go out of business. Over-the-counter drugs tend to be much less active. They fill the need people have to medicate themselves. They do less harm. I guess that's the way I rationalize it," Jim admitted.

"What does the Rule company want of you?"

"With all the publicity headache remedies are getting lately in connection with kidney damage from overuse, they want advice regarding their formulation."

"Doesn't that tend to belie your rationalization?"

"Yes and no," Jim replied. "The folks who get the kidney damage take tremendous amounts daily for years. They clearly abuse the stuff." He paused and then spoke almost to himself. "I'll grant my reasoning seems illogical, but this is a chance to pick up a few thousand bucks with little effort and we may well need it. I guess that's the real reason. Besides, I won't advise them to do anything which would make their product less safe."

"What happens to your objectivity if you are paid by a drug company?"

"What's your problem? Don't you want some more money?"

"Answer the question," Janet demanded with a laugh.

"Objectivity, like specificity, is greatly to be desired but seldom achieved."

"What in hell does that mean?"

"It means," said Jim with a sigh, "that no drug is ever completely free of contamination by other chemicals which may alter it's actions and similarly no matter how hard we may try, factors unrelated to a problem always influence our thoughts about the problem. When I was a student, I was taught that medicines which contained a mixture of drugs were bad. They contained fixed ratios of drugs which the physician could not alter. The right way to administer drugs was to give each one separately in the amount you wanted for your patient which, incidentally, is often less expensive than the mixtures the drug companies market. That argument made sense. Who needs a mixture of aspirin, phenacetin and caffeine? Why not take aspirin alone. Now that I'm being offered compensation from Rule, I've been thinking that APC powders aren't too bad. They seem useful if only for their placebo effect."

"Their what effect?"

"Placebo, a sugar pill, an inert substance that fills your need to treat yourself. Anyhow, since Rule is willing to pay me, I find my position toward their mixture has become more accepting."

"Are you saying aspirin stops headaches psychologically?"

"Sometimes, though studies do show that adequate doses are pain killing. What I am saying is that to some degree money always corrupts, and I'm going to let Rule corrupt me a wee bit. Now lets make love or go to sleep."

"Go to sleep."

"But you've got me wide awake." He slid his arm under his wife and while he probed he kissed her neck, face and whatever exposed skin he could locate.

"Oh what the hell," she replied with a deep sigh and began responding appropriately."

For forty years Charlie Evans had been in the Anatomy department at Wilder. A full professor, he was the faculty member with the longest tenure in the school, having joined as an instructor after completing his doctorate at the age of twenty-four. He hated the thought of mandatory retirement at age sixty-five. Fortunate in that Anatomy was taught first when medical students are still enthusiastic, his contact with them was a never-ending source of pleasure. He seldom lectured, preferring instead to use the Socratic method. On the daily rounds of his students in their dissecting rooms, he constantly questioned them and aided their understanding of the structure of the body relating what they were learning to medical and surgical problems they would later encounter. His enthusiasm and love of teaching were sensed by the students who inevitably grew to love him as a teacher and a man. He was a truly gentle man and no one could remember a time when he had appeared angry or disagreeable.

As he made his rounds he found himself reminiscing more and more of late. He recalled his own introduction to the dissecting room with its penetrating odor of formaldehyde and the wizened human cadavers lying in shallow tanks awaiting their student dissectors. He was horrified as he remembered the old peddler with a basket of candies slung on his shoulder who appeared on the first day and made no sales. Within the week most were buying his wares and setting them on the bodies for later consumption.

He remembered, too, the two girls in his class who dumped cheap perfume in their cadaver's tank in a misguided attempt to improve the smell. The resulting smell was so much worse than the original that even the instructors refused to enter their dissecting area and all their practical examinations had to be taken on someone else's cadaver.

Charlie had many happy memories, but soon he might be leaving. He hoped desperately he would be allowed to stay on and teach. Though his retirement was mandatory, he could teach through age seventy with yearly appointments if the new head approved. That selection process would begin next fall, and probably be similar to the choosing of a head for Pharmacology in which he was presently engaged. He hoped the Pharmacology choice would go smoothly and that he could survive the procedure without making anyone angry—anyone powerful at least. He recognized Block and Shane as the two members of the committee who wielded the most influence, and they were the two he felt least sympathetic toward. Larry Root, of Bacteriology, was a pompous ass, but he had always managed to get along with him. Tatum and Kulp were younger and not apt to be problems. John Block had already let him know, through a series of hints, that when it came to a vote he had better see thing Block's way so that he, Block, could ensure a sympathetic new head for Anatomy. Charlie wasn't certain just how much Block could influence that choice, but he suspected Block was not bluffing.

He was engaged in such speculation when his attention was aroused by loud raucous laughter coming from one of the nearby dissecting rooms. He noticed a red-faced, female student, half-running, half-walking down the hall toward him. She stared straight ahead, avoided his questioning glances, and left the Anatomy dissecting rooms clearly upset. Charlie was familiar with this student as she was both self assured and beautiful. He guessed she might be the top student in the class.

As the incident had begun with laughter, he suspected that nothing serious had happened, but was curious to learn the origin of her discomfort. He wondered to which of the student pranks this student had fallen victim. Sauntering into the dissecting room from which the girl had come, he spied one of the male students admiring what appeared to be his cadaver's amputated penis. Since amputation can hardly be considered useful dissection, Charlie could feel himself starting to anger. The students noticed his strange look and fell silent. Before reacting, Charlie glanced at the cadaver and noted a properly dissected penis in place.

"Where did that come from?" he asked with genuine curiosity.

"There," the student answered pointing to the cadaver and proudly handing the object in his hand to Charlie.

The usual penile dissection begins with the removal of the skin to reveal the anatomy beneath. The dissector of this organ had taken extreme pains to remove the outer skin by peeling it from the lower abdomen as one sometimes removes a tight sock: pulling it inside out. Someone had then filled the void in the righted skin with a tightly rolled wad of paper towels.

Charlie nodded. "Very clever," he admitted. "How did you manage to upset Miss Nugent with that?"

The student, noting Charlie's usual friendliness returning, warmed to the explanation. "We've invented a game we play, Dr. Evens. One of us is given an organ or part of an organ behind our back. We're supposed to identify it by feel. Today was Dorothy's turn, and we prepared that specimen for her. You should have been here to watch her face as she tried to tell us what it was. It was a riot."

"No doubt you all tried to help her with hints and remarks," Charlie observed dryly.

"Certainly. She's such a darn good student it was fascinating to see her at a loss for words. She never did even guess."

Another student gleefully added, "She gave up and finally admitted defeat—then dropped it like a hot potato when she saw what it was." The group started laughing again.

"Are you all prepared for a quiz on that dissection?" Charlie asked. The laughter subsided and the students returned to their dissections.

"Let me know when you are," Charlie remarked and turned and left the room.

Two gleaming stainless steel tables stood on the terrazzo floor of the autopsy room. Each was eight feet long by four feet wide. At one end, a sink was incorporated into the table. A water tap ran continuously to aid the pathologist in cleaning body organs or sucking fluids from the body cavities. The suction apparatus made periodic disgusting sounds similar to a patient with post nasal drip and did little to improve the ambience. No matter how many postmortems Dr. Harry Tatum would take part in, he would never feel truly at ease.

An autopsy is like a puzzle. First, the patient's chart is studied. Here the pathologist has access to the doctor's notes, the laboratory and x-ray data and any other evidence collected prior to the patient's demise. With large knives, scissors and bone saws, the pathologist exposes the silent subject's inner workings and views them. Sometimes telltale signs of this or that disorder may be seen by the unaided eye or noted by the nose. Often, signs appear when the organs are sliced and small portions run through the gamut of solutions, techniques and stains which result in the colorful hair-thin sections pathologists study under their microscopes. When all these data are assembled, a picture of the patient's disorder may emerge.

As one cynical professor used to remark, "Doctors take great pride in seeing their diagnoses confirmed at autopsy." The corollary to that remark is certainly true. At autopsy, no clinician likes to learn he has missed the diagnosis especially if the cause of death were treatable.

Today's autopsy was an unhappy one. The subject, Billy Owens, had hardly begun to live. The students in attendance were stunned to see how beautiful was this six-months-old dead child. The waste could not have been more forcefully dramatized. Billy's parents must have been devastated.

Dr. Tatum showed the babies organs to the assembled group. They were mostly fresh and healthy looking. In dissecting a fresh as opposed to an embalmed body, the beauty of the smooth, glistening and colorful surfaces of the organs encountered is striking.

When he came to the abdominal cavity, Dr. Tatum worked very carefully. The pediatricians had suspected an intestinal intussuseception.

An intestinal intussuseception is a telescoping of the intestine into itself. When this occurs, the blood vessels which supply the intestinal wall from the outside are caught between the outer surfaces of the intestine which reflect upon themselves and are compressed. The blood supply is thus compromised and gangrenous areas of the intestines are formed. Uncorrected, death can occur in forty-eight hours.

In this case the baby was described as "colicky", and one day passed before the seriousness of the situation was even faintly suspected. A series of unfortunate errors ensued which finalized with the lamentable result before them.

"Here is the culprit." Harry drew apart the cut abdominal walls with his gloved hands and moved his head, neck and shoulders to the side exposing the child's innards to the assembled students. He motioned toward a curved sausage-like portion of the discolored intestine with a twist of his head. "You can see the difference in color from the remainder of the intestine. He stared directly at one of the students. "Brown," he asked, "is this a typical-aged child to be suspicious of this condition?"

Terry Brown answered, "yes, sir. I believe these occur mostly in the first two years of life and are more common in boys."

"Are these difficult to diagnose?" the doctor asked.

Terry hesitated. "I wouldn't have thought so, but this one must have been missed, so I guess it can be."

"It depends on where in the intestine they occur," Dr. Tatum announced. "I don't know why this wasn't recognized and reduced surgically. If caught in time, there isn't too much to the treatment." He went on lecturing and questioning the students as he completed the autopsy. He dismissed the students, washed up and got back into his street clothes feeling depressed about the youngster he should never have seen had not some unfortunate set of circumstances come together to produce the tragedy. He was torn between wanting to ferret out the reasons and assigning blame, and truly not wanting to know how it had happened.

Harry was softhearted. He liked to be nice to people, and he was caught. If some resident or intern were guilty of negligence in this case, wouldn't the result alone be the strongest punishment he or she could receive? Yet, when he thought of the child's parents, did they not deserve that such negligence would not go unpunished? Or were they the negligent ones? Harry felt uncomfortable. He had better get to the bottom of this case quickly.

Back in his office, he reviewed the chart very carefully. The child was seen at the Wilder Hospital emergency room two days before he died. The first note made much of the child's past history of colic and his fretful parents and implied the fretfulness caused the colic. Harry recognized the house officer's signature as that of one who was headed for a residency in psychiatry and was dismayed by the thought that the quality of medicine practiced by that group was so poor. He had known some good clinicians in that field; but, all too often, the troubled and less gifted in medical school classes drifted into that specialty. He noted that the child was sent home, a four hour drive to the mountains, with sedation and some medicine to relieve the colic.

An unlucky circumstance not appearing in the chart, but which Harry later uncovered talking with the house staff in Pediatrics, played a significant role. Fred Price, the intern who saw the child in the emergency room Saturday morning, was starting an affair with the pediatrics resident-on-call that weekend. In order to keep the way clear for his potential conquest, he was thoughtfully attempting to lighten her clinical load. He should have called for a pediatric consult that Saturday morning instead of prescribing sedatives.

The Owens family went home. At first, the sedation quieted the baby, but the persistence of the condition led his parents to seek aid in a nearer private hospital. The Owens were neither affluent nor insured, and were advised to return to Wilder, part of the system of state supported hospitals. They became frantic trying to quiet the baby and used more and more of the medicines they had been given. When they arrived again at the emergency room late Sunday, the child, who was now drugged, appeared to be sleeping peacefully. The nurse on duty called Dr. Price. On hearing the child was quiet and asleep, he went back to his carnal pursuits and let the matter literally sit in the emergency room. By the time someone recognized the difference between terminal coma and peaceful sleep, it was too late.

When Harry finished the report of his autopsy findings, which contained none of Freddie Price's peccadilloes, he was certain the puzzle had been solved. His curiosity about this case had been satisfied though he regretted looking into it. It was the responsibility of the Pediatrics Department to air the manner in which this child's death could have been avoided. His responsibility was limited to determining exactly what had happened; not why.

As he was mulling over the tragedy, he suddenly recalled a conversation he had had with Jim Kulp several years earlier concerning Freddie Price then a second-year medical student. Harry remembered Jim's saying, "If I could personally put a student out of school, Fred Price would go. He may pass examinations, but he's shown me a complete lack of effort in the laboratory exercises. If he's that lazy in the student lab why should he be conscientious in his clinical duties?"

Others, too, had noted that Freddie Price as marginal in his concern for patients; yet he was smart enough to pass examinations and soon would finish his residency at Wilder and be gone. Though he would personally never use or recommend Dr. Price as a physician, Harry Tatum wasn't about to rock the boat by proposing an investigation of Billy Owens' case.

Several days later Harry Tatum met with John Block and Marge Sparrow, Dr. Block's technician, in the animal quarters.

"Dr. Block," Marge insisted, "there is no mistake. Those three drugs are made up in the same strength solutions and administered in the same dose by stomach tube as you told me."

"Could you be killing them with the stomach tube?" Harry asked Marge.

"Not likely," John interjected. "Marge has stomach tubed rats for years. There must be some other explanation." He drummed his fingers on a laboratory table where the drug solutions stood in flasks.

"We won't get to go the full ten weeks if the aspirin and acetaminophen rats continue to die. The survivors in those groups don't look well to me," Harry observed. "The phenacetin rats look great. Maybe they'll survive ten weeks."

John nodded in agreement. "We may still show the kidney damage with the phenacetin treated rats," he said. "I was never too keen about those other groups. Peter Markley suggested them. He felt it would make a better experiment."

"Why?" Harry asked.

John sighed. "Peter still feels aspirin may be the culprit," he explained, "and as acetaminophen is the substance phenacetin is converted into in the body and is currently being marketed as Tylenol which is rapidly gaining in popularity as an over-the-counter headache remedy, he felt we should include it."

"Dr. Block," Marge asked, "do you want me to autopsy rats which die before the ten week period of drug administration? The protocol you gave me does not call for that."

John turned to Harry. "I wanted a nice clean experiment. I anticipated all the animals would live and did not want us to autopsy rats whose tissues weren't obtained quickly after death. Since the phenacetin group seems okay so far and that's the group I want to show the kidney damage with, I don't see why we should bother with those others that die." He stared at Harry and seeing no reaction, he addressed his technician. "No, Marge, if the aspirin and Tylenol rats continue to die, and I suspect they will, we'll just abandon that part of the study and concentrate our efforts the phenacetin-treated rats."

Harry remained silent as John's tone had left no doubt that he had made up his mind. Harry was curious as to why the rats were dying, but he had plenty of other things to do and was not about to argue with John though his instincts told him this was poor Science.

"Marge," John ordered, "keep me informed. If the phenacetin animals seem to be getting sick we can always reduce the dose. As long as they do okay we'll keep things as they are. See anything wrong with that, Harry?" he asked offhandedly.

"Not if you're bent on producing a kidney lesion with phenacetin," Harry answered.

John nodded. "That's what I'm determined to do," he said flatly.

Twelve miles away, in the city of Chester, Jim Kulp was entering the brick building which housed the Rule Pharmaceutical Company. Several offices and a single laboratory were in the front of the building while a manufacturing plant and shipping decks took up the back. The building was old—quite unlike the gleaming edifices which constitute much of the wealthy ethical drug industry.

Jim was ushered into the office of Reggie Pate, the president. Reggie had worked as a boy in old Doc Rule's family drugstore in Chester. He had jerked sodas and been a general helper. Doc Rule had liked Reggie and sent him to pharmacy school. Reggie stayed with Doc and eventually took over the running of all his business interests as time enfeebled the older man. Now Reggie was approaching retirement. Recent developments suggesting his main product, a headache powder, might be causing medical problems disturbed him. His company was even becoming involved in law suits. He clearly needed some help. Inquiries had been made at Wilder for someone who might be able to advise him and Jim Kulp's name had come to him through a mutual acquaintance.

Reggie's large office was dominated by his mahogany desk at it's center. The oak paneled walls lent a quiet dignity to the surroundings. In the office with Reggie, sat Bill Anderson, Rule's vice president and chief financial officer. He had joined Reggie to run the financial side of the business. Reggie was tall, thin, wiry and gray. He had a twinkle in his eye and the ghost of a smile ever present in his expression. By contrast, Mr. Anderson was short, stocky, blond, young and very serious.

After introductions had been made, Reggie thanked Jim for coming. "I thought we ought to get to know each other," he said, "discuss what we'd like you to do for us, and then go to the club for lunch if you can spare the time?"

"Sounds great, I'd enjoy that," said Jim, who, not knowing what to expect, had set aside most of the day for this meeting.

Reggie started by telling Jim the history of the product, Doc Rule and the Company. From time to time, Mr. Anderson would add something and Jim sensed that Reggie resented these interruptions. Reggie began calling Jim "Doc," and Jim had the feeling that his own respectful silence was endearing him to the man.

"What do you know about Rule's Powders?" Reggie asked.

"Just that they're a powder form of an APC," Jim answered.

"Ever take them?" the old man asked.

"No."

"Miss Rankin," Reggie called his secretary. "Have Alfred make up a package of powders for Dr. Kulp, please. Once you have tried them, you'll prefer them to tablets," he said, returning to Jim.

Jim smiled. "If I'm going to work for you I should know what they're like," he said.

"By the way," Reggie asked, "what do you charge for your services?"

"I really don't know," said Jim, "I've never consulted before."

Reggie's face lost expression and he eyed Jim for several seconds. Slowly his smile reappeared. "Would one hundred dollars a day be reasonable?"

Jim was paid a salary by the University and was allowed some consulting which was pertinent to his field. Any fees were a windfall. Reggie's offer seemed generous. "Seems fine," he answered.

"Good," Reggie said with a smile and a quick glance at his vice president. "The spot we're in at the moment is this. The government is about to require us to print a warning on our product that it may cause kidney trouble because it contains phenacetin. What do you think about that?"

"Pinning the blame on phenacetin is premature," Jim answered, "but there seems little doubt that overuse of these analgesic preparations seems to produce kidney problems."

"Well we don't want the warning on the product, so we're considering removing the phenacetin. Can you suggest a substitute?" Reggie asked.

"Why bother with a substitute? Just increase the dose of aspirin," Jim suggested. "That will give you an equivalent amount of pain-killing and I doubt anyone could tell the difference unless the taste is changed."

"Most of the taste is produced by the salt filler," Bill Anderson interjected.

Reggie cocked his head. "You don't think customers could tell if we removed phenacetin and added more aspirin?" he asked.

"I really don't, sir," Jim answered.

"We could test market some in a small area," Bill Anderson suggested. Reggie shot Bill one of his expressionless looks and returned to Jim. "Doc, what about replacing the phenacetin with salicylamide?"

"There's not much evidence that drug does anything, but it doesn't seem to be harmful. I guess you could put it in if you really want to," Jim said.

"What would you do, Doc?" Reggie asked.

"I wouldn't change the present formulation."

"What about that damned warning?" Reggie persisted.

"I don't believe anyone will even notice it," Jim answered. "If they do, I doubt it will bother them." He was thinking about the present warnings on these preparations which tell patients to take limited amounts and see their doctor if the headaches persist. The patients who end up with kidney lesions certainly didn't heed those warnings.

"We don't want a warning about phenacetin on our powders," Reggie said with finality. "We'll have to remove it." After a few seconds of thought, he added, "How about some lunch, Doc? You hungry?"

"I can always eat, sir," Jim admitted with a grin.

They lunched at a businessman's eating club in a Chester hotel. Reggie knew everyone and was obviously a well liked and respected member of the Chester business community. He introduced Jim to more people than Jim could ever remember and gave him the feeling of being part of a large "in group" which Jim did not normally have. His lunches were usually eaten at his desk or in the departmental library from a paper bag brought from home. Another function of the eating club was the serving of alcoholic beverages which public restaurants were forbidden by law. Between the alcohol, the pleasant surroundings, the delicious lunch and the feeling that Reggie liked him, Jim was thoroughly enjoying his first venture into the industrial arena.

During lunch, Jim began to expound on the difficulties involved in demonstrating the analgesic action of a drug. "Painkilling is the very devil to measure," he pointed out. "Pain is hard to measure. I can't feel yours, you cant feel mine."

"You don't appear to feel any pain," Bill Anderson quipped noting Jim's suddenly expansive mood.

Jim grinned self-consciously. "I'm not used to cocktails at lunch," he admitted.

"Hell, Doc, don't pay any attention to this glorified accountant," Reggie said with a disapproving glance at their luncheon companion. "Go on with your thoughts."

Bill Anderson again looked grave, his one attempt at humor having fared badly.

"Pain is purely subjective," Jim continued. "We can measure responses to pain-producing stimuli in animals, but we aren't sure it is pain they're feeling. We assume it is pain because we find the same stimuli painful or uncomfortable. We say 'it burns, it pinches, it's sharp,' but we don't know what an animal feels. You really have to test these drugs in man, and that process isn't easy. Sugar pills have produced relief from pain associated with surgery in seventy percent of patients in some studies. That doesn't leave much room for improvement by an active drug."

Reggie had listened attentively. "What you're saying, Doc, is that it is hard to prove our product works."

"Or doesn't work," Bill Anderson added.

"Exactly, sir, but don't sell short the fact that people continue to use it. 'You can fool some of the people some of the time.' There's some damn good evidence that aspirin relieves pain. It's dose related. The more aspirin the more pain relief."

Luncheon drew to a close with pecan pie, a rich specialty of the house. Jim went back to Wilder bearing a large supply of Rule's headache powders and the feeling he had a new friend in Reggie Pate.

Dr. Lawrence James Root, M.D., Ph.D., a full professor, held a joint appointment in Bacteriology and Medicine and was a member of the hospitals infectious disease team. An impressive looking man with thick gray hair and a large frame. He moved slowly and deliberately, and the quickest thing about him was his easily provoked temper. He was totally devoid of humor and thus tended toward pomposity. He fully intended to replace Frank Mackenzie as Dean of the Medical School when Frank retired, and signs and rumors that another was being groomed for that position had been disturbing to him even though he tended to discount such absurdities.

The infectious disease team consisted of a group of clinicians who were interested primarily in diseases caused by infectious organisms. Their function was to determine as quickly as possible which agents were causing the trouble and how best to eradicate them without harming the patient. Since infectious diseases can move with startling rapidity and the choice of the proper therapeutic agent requires a combination of skills in Bacteriology, Pharmacology, Medicine and occasionally Surgery many hospitals field such a team, in recognition that several heads are usually better than one.

Professor Root was sitting in his office in the Bacteriology Department reading when a knock on his door produced a pained expression on his face. "Who is it?" he groaned.

"It is me, Daniel, may I talk with you?" a relatively soft voice answered. Daniel Pope, Ph.D. headed the Bacteriology Department. He was the antithesis of Professor Root. He was sparely built, balding, and full of good humor. He found Root an annoyance and had hoped for years that he would be offered a head ship somewhere else; anywhere.

"Come in. Dr. Pope." Root rose from his chair and opened the door. "To what do I owe this unexpected pleasure?"

Dr. Pope thought, Thank God he's in a good mood. He said, "I need to see you about some administrative matters."

Root motioned Dr. Pope toward a chair and they faced each other across Root's desk. Root slowly lit his pipe.

Why does he always seem to make me feel at a disadvantage, thought Dr. Pope. I'm the department head. "Larry, Dean Mackenzie wants those of us who have grants to take summer salary." he announced.

"What's that?" Dr. Root mumbled puffing on his pipe.

"Our salaries, though paid monthly, are actually based on a nine month school year. You could go off for the three summer months and do something else if you weren't in Medicine too."

"I've noticed several of you old timers in the basic sciences doing just that."

Dr. Pope ignored Root's intended slur. "It's a throwback to when Wilder was a two-year school. Anyhow, through a technicality, the University pays on the basis of nine months. Since you work all summer in research, you can take those months three-twelfths or one-fourth, out of your grant. You, in essence, get a twenty-five percent pay raise."

"You mean it goes on top of my present salary?"

"Yes."

"Hmm, but I didn't put salary for myself as an item in my grant application."

"You'll have to do it in your grant renewals, but you apparently do not need to have applied for it. Just as long as you have unexpended funds, you can draw summer salary. The Dean's office has been in contact with Washington and it's okay."

"Sounds crazy to me."

"I couldn't agree more, Larry," Dr. Pope answered "It means anyone in this school who has National Institutes of Health Research Grants can give himself a twenty-five percent raise if he has the funds."

"My funds are fairly well earmarked for the research I'm doing."

"Then you won't get a raise," said Dan with subdued glee.

Professor Root sat puffing his pipe for some seconds. "Can I use money budgeted for equipment?"

"It is my understanding any unexpended funds in your grant can be used."

"That is crazy. It is like saying there's money on the floor. If you want it pick it up. I did want a recording spectrophotoflurometer for the laboratory and have it budgeted. I wonder if I really need it."

"That is a choice you will have to make," Dr. Pope smiled. He already has, he thought.

"How do I go about getting this done?"

"When you've decided, just let me know and I will see the paperwork is taken care of by my secretary." He rose to go. "How is the search progressing?"

"We're waiting for replies from the inquiries we've sent." It was clear Professor Roots thoughts were elsewhere.

He's probably figuring what he'll do with his windfall and without his instrument, Dr. Pope chuckled to himself as he left.

In fact, Lawrence Root was thinking much loftier thoughts. He was considering how the monies the government was spending on medical research had influenced the direction medical education and research were taking. Positioned between the basic and clinical sciences, he had noted the rapidity with which the changes were coming. It was harder and harder to get good graduate students into the basic sciences. A student could get his M.D., go into a clinical department and do the same research a basic scientist would do, and receive twice the salary. In the past, the clinical departments spent most of their efforts caring for patients and doing small amounts of clinical research. Basic research in a clinical department was practically unheard of. Now that lots of funds for research were available many of the clinical departments did "Basic research." The obtaining of grant monies was becoming more important than patient care. The doctor who was interested primarily in caring for his patients and teaching students to do the same was considered second-rate. Publications and a national image were what was required for fame and fortune. In many departments, junior members brought in more money through grants than the department head obtained through the departmental budget. He was thus becoming impotent. Many thought of the head as a janitor who kept the place running smoothly for their benefit. Many deans exploited this situation, feeling their own power was best served by keeping the troublesome on their faculty warring amongst themselves.

This salary supplements from grants, thought Root, gave the Dean a way to build up a state school without having to obtain the funds from the state legislature.

The Dean could eventually become a powerful figure in the state. He'd like that.

When his mind returned to his local surroundings, he noted he was alone. Funny, he couldn't recall Dan's leaving. Such an unprepossessing man to head his department. It was almost embarrassing.

"Rod. why don't we go somewhere this weekend? Mary's old enough to take care of the kids now. They'd enjoy it and Lord knows we deserve some time to ourselves." Marie Barret came as close to pleading with her husband as she was able.

Rodney was thinking of all the work he had to do and, under ordinary circumstances, would have said so. Yet, under ordinary circumstances he would not have had to say so—Marie would never have made such a request. It was becoming painfully apparent to him just how selfish a life he had led. Under his drive to become a successful researcher, he had let Marie and the family sacrifice so much. Now her illness brought into focus the reality of their relationship. He had allowed Marie to make all the adjustments and now her condition was requiring efforts on his part. Was he really ready and willing to make the efforts to help her?

Following Linda Koster's visit he had finally faced the truth concerning the seriousness of his wife's condition. As an abstract medical problem, he had immediately found it interesting. Any biologist would. What happens to an organism when you block the functions of a major excretory system? How can you bypass the blockade so that the organism may live? These were fascinating questions worthy of the time of any investigator. When they were no longer abstract; but applied to a member of your family, especially your wife, the shoe was on a different foot. He found it very hard to accept Marie's condition; for when he did, he gave her up for dead. She might last for days, months, years, even decades; but her course was downhill and that prospect, for a loved one, is hard to face. In the past, Marie had been his strength, part of his drive and ambition. It wasn't that he lacked these, he didn't; but their combined strengths were formidable. She had helped him through graduate school where he had excelled. She helped him at Wilder, and his research for such a young investigator had given him a high degree of national prominence in his field. He could not imagine life without her, yet life with her was not the same. She now required his help and this interfered with his work as he had done it in the past. In the cold logic of biology, she had become a less useful appendage he should amputate for the good of the cause. He was immediately struck with guilt and was thankful that such thoughts are deep in one's mind and seldom see the light of day.

"Where would you like to go?" he finally asked.

"Why not the mountains? They can be lovely this time of year. We could go up to the parkway and drive south on it."

"Is it open? It snows in the mountains in February, you know."

"I'll call that inn where we stayed last summer," she answered clearly getting excited and more animated than Rodney had seen her in months. "We could leave Friday night after my dialysis, and we wouldn't have to be back until Sunday night. It would be like another honeymoon."

God knows I could use that, he thought. "That would be nice," he said.

No snow blocked the parkway, the inn had room, and the Barrets had a second honeymoon. Unlike the first, Marie lacked sexual drive and Rodney, with enough for both of them, was inhibited by Marie's impossible to disguise reluctance. They both spent too much time apologizing and feeling sorry for each other and themselves. The weekend was depressing; contrasting so vividly their past life with their present. A time on the way to the inn the majestic views of the mountains elevated their moods. That elevation was replaced by considerations of fluid intake, diet selection, odors of certain molecules which when not excreted by the kidneys appear on the skin and the ever present reminder in the form of access tubing. It takes a truly mature and unselfish love to transcend those considerations.

They both wanted Rodney to be the new Head of Pharmacology and that challenge both helped and hindered their relationship. It gave them a purpose which helped lessen their attention to their personal problems, but it required Rodney's time and so did Marie.

Reggie Pate stood at his office window looking out at the roof tops of Chester. His right hand was stroking his chin and his left hand was supporting his right elbow. The view before him was not a spectacular one as views go, but it didn't matter as Reggie was unaware of his optic nerve impulses. He was in deep thought and he was frustrated. The headache powders his firm marketed sold well in the Southeast and profits were good, but they were fast being threatened by those damned idiotic legal suits which were appearing with increasing frequency. Plaintiffs were seeking higher and higher damages and this last legal case was asking for millions. He couldn't afford to employ full-time legal talent, and the necessary retainers and legal fees were becoming prohibitive as was the insurance. What piqued him most was what he considered the unfairness of the situation. Rarely had he known of any harm coming from sensible use of the product; occasional hangovers and headaches. You weren't supposed to make a steady diet of them. It clearly warned against excess usage on the package. "If only the powders were used in moderation," he whispered to himself.

What would happen to the profits then? A recess of his brain, instantly queried and answered, was quickly suppressed. A buzzer sounded and Reggie walked to his desk and pressed the lever on his communications system. His secretary's voice came through.

"Mr. Brandon is here."

"Send him in, please, Miss Rankin." He started toward the door.

Roger Brandon practically bounced into the room. His immaculate sartorial state and efficient manner clearly indicated success. "Hello, Reggie, I'm glad to see you."

Reggie had known and done business with Roger's father, also a lawyer. Fees and cases were fewer and less expensive then. His father had been a gentler and more soothing person to deal with for Reggie, and he would never get used to being called "Reggie" by this forty-year-old kid. He grudgingly employed him because he was the best local attorney and he felt out of towners were at a disadvantage in local jury trials.

"Roger, where do you stand in this Johnson case? Does she really expect to get two million five?"

"That's what they're asking, Reg." Roger's enthusiastic bounce had now modulated to the undertaker-like seriousness that told Reggie the meter was running. At such time he didn't feel comfortable taking the time to resent being called by his first name. Sensing Reggie's discomfort, Roger continued confidently.

"I'm sure we can get by for comfortably less. We can stall them into a settlement."

Sure, drag it out forever and collect bigger fees, thought Reggie. He shrugged. "I'd like to see it settled, but if we could win one of these and set a precedent so we wouldn't be constantly harassed by these suits..." His voice trailed off as he stood in deep thought. Suddenly he became imbued with an optimism he had not previously shown. "I want to go to the wire on this one, Roger. Let's win this case and put a stop to this nonsense."

"I don't know, Reg. This case may be tougher to win than most, and so far all have been settled."

"But this one is a pharmacist. Pharmacists should know better."

Perhaps, but she is also a Negro and if you dig your heels in on this one you're apt to be called a bigot."

Reggie glared at Roger. "Hell, it wouldn't be the first time. Black, red, yellow, what difference? If they're wrong, they're wrong!"

"It's the jury we're up against. The poor slob wronged by the rich company. You know the lyrics by now, Reg."

Reggie snorted. "I know, but let's put up one hell of a fight and discourage this trend. I want you to get together with Dr. Jim Kulp from Wilder Medical School. Between the two of you with all your fancy titles and degrees you ought to be able to come up with something." He looked expectantly at Roger Brandon hoping for some encouraging sign.

"I'll be glad to meet with the good doctor, but unless he's a genius I wouldn't hope for much. These suits are just a part of the cost of doing business."

Reggie exploded. "Too damned big a cost! I may have to seek less expensive legal aid," he said pointedly.

"And settle for more with the plaintiffs," Roger shot back with a smile.

"If they're really that damaged, I'd a hell of a lot sooner see them get it than you legal eagles."

The smile vanished from Roger's face, but Reggie hardly noticed."

"Miss Rankin," he called into his communicator, "please get Dr. Kulp on the phone." He turned to Roger. "When would you find it possible to met with Jim?"

One week later Jim Kulp visited the opulent offices of Brandon and McCollum in the Chester Bank building. As most of his time was spent in unprepossessing laboratory surroundings or relatively dingy classrooms, he was impressed by the trappings of a financially successful law practice. As he waited in the large outer office he could not help but note the pulchritudinous secretaries busily filling large clean white sheets of paper with mysterious dark lines of letters signifying lord knows what information of import. The importance he took for granted, else how could these partners afford these surroundings. He was musing thus when Roger Brandon strode toward him, hand stretched out in greeting, and following his self-introduction escorted him back to his private office. Jim observed as he passed Roger's private secretary in a room of her own between the outer and inner office that a definite prerequisite for employment here must be a pretty face and trim figure. He jokingly voiced his thought and Roger, with no hint of humor, made reference to his own personal propensity to go "first class." They went quickly to the business at hand.

"Mrs. Johnson is a pharmacist. She and her husband own their own drugstore in the Negro section of Chester. Last year she developed kidney failure and had to go on dialysis. Her condition has become permanent and she'll require dialysis for the rest of her life. Her personal physician ascribes her troubles to her intake of APC powders, and she's suing Rule Pharmaceutical Company for selling her this dangerous product. She's asking two point five million dollars in the aggregate."

Jim whistled. "That's a lot. What are her chances of winning?"

"Ordinarily we'd probably settle for one-tenth that amount after a suitable period of negotiations, but Reggie wants to fight this one and try to set a precedent. If it goes to a jury, anything can happen."

"But no one knows for sure the powders are truly responsible for kidney disease."

"You mean there is no evidence that these drugs hurt the kidney?" Roger asked pointedly.

"I mean there is no clear-cut evidence."

"But your medical literature speaks of the 'phenacetin lesion'." Roger stressed the word "your".

"True, but the concept is not universally excepted. There are investigators who are sold on it, but many are not."

"Unfortunately we can't wait around for you scientists to make up your minds. We're in the real world and have to work with what we have. Mrs. Johnson's attorney will employ some expert who will testify that Reggie's product is the proximate cause of her problems. Would you be willing to testify that it isn't?"

Jim was slow to answer. He wanted to help Reggie as he believed these suits were unwarranted, but he had no desire to testify. "I don't think I'd make a good witness. I'm not well known in this field scientifically, and I'm not involved in treating patients, but I might be able to find you an expert to testify."

Roger looked appraisingly at Jim and wondered why Reggie had bothered to suggest their getting together.

Jim continued. "Besides, I don't think the question of whether the powders are causing the kidney lesion is important to the issue."

Rogers flagging interest was renewed. "How so?" he inquired.

"With present state of our scientific knowledge, you can't prove that the powders didn't cause the trouble, but everyone in the field seems to agree that you have to take one hell of a lot of these to cause problems; far in excess of recommended amounts. If we concede they caused the problem, we can claim the product was abused. Is abuse the manufacturer's problem?"

Roger temporarily ignored the question but was obviously considering Jim's approach. It was not a new strategy to him. He had thought about it previously. The directions on the package warned the user to see his physician if the headaches persisted and not to take more than four powders a day. The sort of dosage that was thought to produce these kidney problems was more like ten to twenty powders a day for a like number of years. Jim was right that did constitute abuse of the product, but "abuse" is a difficult concept to sell a jury bent on helping a poor plaintiff against a big bad wealthy company. He finally spoke. "What we need if we use that strategy is a clear presentation which would impress any jury that the user, not the manufacturer, is at fault. I'm not at all sure we could pull it off."

"What can I do to help, other than testifying?"

"Let me give you copies of all the depositions and records in this case. Study them and see what you can come up with that would emphasize that Mrs. Johnson and not the Rule Pharmaceutical Company is to blame for her troubles. Maybe you can help. As it is, I've advised Reggie to settle out of court. I still consider that good advice."

Jim left the office with an armful of paper. He was intrigued with the idea of contributing to the solution of this problem. After all, research is problem solving.

He remembered that as an undergraduate college student he had rejected the law because he did not think quibbling was a worthy profession. Now as he thought of suggesting ways out of this dilemma, and seeing his suggestions actually used in court to solve the problem, was appealing. Then too, he was being paid for his efforts. This recompense was a tangible form of flattery of which he was much in need.

The medical school library was well used. Though its uses were varied and included naps by exhausted house staff or sleepy students, and even sexual encounters in the far recesses of stacks of books and journals which spanned several floors, the mass of information and misinformation housed there was too huge for human comprehension. It took a staff of several full-time librarians and many part-time student helpers to keep the place in order. Jim wasn't sure where to begin. He didn't even know exactly what he was searching for—just something which would dramatically demonstrate the ridiculousness of the plaintiffs case. He started his random search by scanning the current medical journals. These as yet unbound magazines contained the latest published studies of human or animal experiments in various medical specialties. These journals are usually collected after a set period of time and sent to a bindery where a particular journal's copies spanning one year's time, for example, may be bound together in a hard-cover volume appropriately labeled with gold leaf. These volumes are then shelved with other years of the same journal in the stacks. Some of the older journals go back to the turn of the century or even before. Since there are in excess of two thousand separate journals, each with many volumes, the finding of a particular piece of information may make the search for "a needle in a haystack" appear simple.

Jim had flipped through the pages of several of the publications in the reading room of the library set aside for current journals. This reading room is most used by the students, interns, residents, and attending physicians attempting to keep up on all the latest developments so as not to be embarrassed by their superiors on ward rounds. A thorough knowledge of the latest therapy for the rarest disease on the wards will often pay bigger dividends in prestige than will information leading to the cure of the more common garden variety of illnesses. As he had found nothing that seemed to be in the least bit helpful, and the presence of so many other readers distracted him, he decided on a different tack. He crossed the hall to a room which housed hard-backed texts of many scientific subjects all concerned with the practice of medicine and scanned the index. His eye caught a promising subject and he quickly turned to a particular page of the book and read rapidly. A broad smile spread across his face as he finished one page and started on the next. He began laughing out loud and his laughter, though subdued, sounded noisy in the hushed library. Odd looks from his few fellow readers made him suddenly self-conscious and uncomfortable. The negative feeling was short-lived, however, as he realized he had found just what he wanted: an example which was closely parallel to the misuse of headache powders causing kidney disease, but which under no circumstance a sane juror could possibly hold the purveyor of the product responsible. He left the library in the good mood that comes with accomplishment of a difficult task—a condition with which he had little experienced of late.

Harry Tatum was very excited. Just thirty minutes had passed since his technician had brought him the tray of slides from the phenacetin rat study. A majority of the rats had survived the huge doses literally rammed down their throats twice daily for ten weeks. Now their kidneys were showing signs of wear. In some, the wear was in the right place and the damage did resemble that seen in humans who seriously overindulged in headache remedies for years on end. John Block would be delighted. They had done it. He carefully reexamined the slides but, to one degree or another all the animals showed kidney damage. He called John who was in his office in a flash and was now sitting at Harry's microscope examining the slides.

"There it is. The phenacetin lesion, by God! They all seem to show it. Every single kidney is damaged. Well, this should settle the argument," John stated triumphantly.

"It's unfortunate we lost our controls," Harry cautiously suggested.

"What do you mean?" John looked sharply at Harry.

"The other groups died," Harry reminded him.

"Do we have any of this same batch of rats that were not treated at all?" John asked.

"I don't know. We might".

"Well, if we have, sacrifice a few and make slides of their kidneys.

That would give us a control that didn't receive phenacetin. You don't think these rats have papillary necrosis normally, do you?" John sounded contemptuous.

"Of course not, John. I've never seen papillary lesions like those in any rats, but a good experiment requires controls." Harry answered.

"Then do what I suggested. I hope we have the rats. If not, order, beg, borrow, or steal some." John's mood was not to be dampened by Harry's caution. "Hell, Harry, we did it. We're the first, unless someone else did it at the same time. We'd better write it up and get off an abstract for the Atlantic City meeting right away."

"But what about the controls?"

"Oh, hell, man, it's got to be the phenacetin. You said yourself you'd never seen such kidney damage in rats. We might miss the boat if we don't move fast. I'll write it up and you run controls. If the controls show similar lesions, we can withdraw the paper before the meeting. After all, we'll get priority from the day the abstract's received. That will show we were first to demonstrate the lesion in animals. We can repeat the experiment with controls for a full-fledged publication."

"That's a good idea," said Harry, clearly impressed with the cleverness of John's approach which protected their time priority and yet allowed them at least to control the experiment more carefully. "What do you intend to say about the other drugs killing the rats?"

"Nothing in this first paper. We can study those later." John was clearly ecstatic and Harry wasn't about to voice his misgivings. After all, John Block was a well known and respected medical researcher. Who was he to question the ethics of what John was about to do? Still, Harry was a collaborator in this work, and it didn't seem quite right to present the data this way. He'd discretely seek someone else's opinion. Jim Kulp's field was drugs, and he had always struck Harry as logical and honest. He was entirely unaware of Jim's new consulting arrangement.

The British Journal of Endocrinology returned Jim Kulp's manuscript on the binding of insulin to glass surfaces with a polite "No thank you." Jim suspected that the letter he had sent with his paper revealing that a similar version had been turned down by an American journal may have had something to do with his rejection. He realized his letter had been a mistake, but he felt a full description of what had previously transpired was only fair and that the work would stand on its own merit. The British editors, he thought would be more intelligent. Now, from their editorial remarks, he wasn't so sure. He assembled Donna and Bill in his office to review the situation and decide how to proceed.

"Why don't they accept this work?" Donna asked.

"He's already told you, Donna. It's a threat to the leaders in this field. It makes their work suspect," Bill Michaelson answered.

"It's more than that, Bill. I've tried very hard to put myself in the editor's place. Part of the trouble is they don't trust my mouse assay. The reason for that is some work I did for Jane Bower of the NIH last year. She wanted me to check a sample for her quickly. We were in the midst of an assay using our best mice. I did her assay with what I had left over. The results were crude with a great deal of variance, but they clearly showed the preparation to have insulin-like activity and that's all she wanted to know. I sent her all the data from those imprecise studies, and she's been skeptical of my assay ever since. Despite the fact I made it clear to those were my worst mice, she's down on the assay. The reason I suspect that may be our problem is that the editors did express a willingness to publish the portion of the paper containing experiments done with the radioactive insulin. They trust that: yet, despite the fact the studies with non-radioactive insulin give similar results, they won't accept them. Jane has got to be influencing them. She's an authority in this field."

"I thought she was a friend," Donna complained.

"She is, but she doesn't seem to comprehend statistics. She just doesn't see it."

"So what do we do?" Bill asked.

Jim sat thinking. "If I'm right," he mused, "and it is the assay they distrust, we'll stick so damned much insulin to surfaces that we'll measure it with an assay they do trust like the one used to test commercial insulin vials, the United States Pharmacopoeia test."

"But doesn't that test requires amounts of insulin millions of times more than we're measuring?" Donna asked.

"And won't that require acres of surface?" Bill added.

"Yes," Jim answered with a grin.

"What do we do, rent an all-glass sky scraper?" Bill continued.

"No, we powder the glass," Jim smugly answered.

"Of course," Bill slapped his forehead. "That will give us acres of surface depending on how finely we powder it. A spoonful will be plenty. Why didn't I think of that?"

"You would have," Jim allowed. "We'll filter a concentrated solution of insulin through the powder, then wash it with water or salt solution till none of the original solution is left, and then stir the powder in our gelatin solution. When we drain off the gelatin it ought to contain enough insulin to convulse mice just as they do in the pharmacopoeia assay. We can even measure the blood sugar in the mice and stop their convulsions with glucose injections. If that won't convince the editors, nothing will."

"We ought to be able to do that in a week or less, shouldn't we Donna?" Bill asked.

Donna nodded.

Bill sprang from the chair in which he sat. "Let's do it!" he shouted. "I think we have everything we need."

Bill and Donna went to the lab encouraged and eager to get started. Jim realized they were going to absurd lengths to prove a point; but if it had to be done, so be it. He returned to his work on an upcoming student lecture, but was interrupted by a knock on his office door.

Harry Tatum entered and sprawled in one of the wooden chairs facing his desk. He was hesitant and had trouble choosing his words. "I've come for some advice, Jim. It's rather a sensitive subject so I'd like your assurance our discussion will go no further."

Jim nodded.

Harry continued. "John Block asked me to collaborate with him in some studies he's doing." He described the work to Jim who sat expressionless as he listened until Harry came to the part about John's planning to ignore the fact that aspirin and acetaminophen killed rats, at doses that phenacetin didn't, in his presentation in Atlantic City.

"Hell, Harry, that's misleading. That's dishonest!" Jim shook his head in amazement.

"John says we don't know enough about those drugs yet. He plans to pursue them further later." Harry added.

"But any study he presents showing phenacetin produces kidney lesions which ignores the facts that similar doses of the other drugs kill the animals would lead one to think phenacetin was the toxic drug when in reality the aspirin rats and the acetaminophen rats die before a lesion was even looked for. They are the toxic drugs. Phenacetin is the safest."

"I agree, Jim; but I don't know what I can do about it," Harry shrugged. "Suppose," he went on, "we had never given those other two. Then there would be nothing wrong with John's approach."

"True, but since you gave all three drugs, you implied some sort of comparison. John can't shelve the data merely because they don't suit his purposes."

"John does as he pleases, You know that, Jim."

"He shouldn't be allowed to distort facts knowingly. Damn it, Harry, that is plain dishonest."

"Well, I came to talk with you because I sort of felt uneasy and I wanted a disinterested point of view. If everyone reacts the way you do…"

"Everyone won't," Jim interrupted. "I am particularly disturbed because of late I've seen some of the practical consequences of just this sort of thing."

Jim then told Harry of his consulting for the Rule Pharmaceutical Company and their decision to remove phenacetin from their product.

"In reality John's experiments suggests they may be removing the wrong drug. Those products contain aspirin too. The thing that makes me mad is that the scientific literature ought to be helpful in making such decisions, not misleading us. John is more interested in pushing his point of view than in learning the truth. Since you've told me of this in confidence, I can't do much about it. I hope you'll push him. You're a collaborator." Jim sounded ominous.

Harry looked pained. "John is powerful. If I can't convince him, I don't know what I can do."

"I'll tell you what I'd do. I'd remove my name from the abstract on any publication I felt was misleading."

Harry looked thoughtful. "I'll try and get him to see things our way, but I won't mention our talk."

When Harry had gone, Jim tried to go back to his lecture, but his mind kept returning to his talk with Harry. The reason he had reacted so strongly was at least partly his recent connection with the Rule Company, yet whether phenacetin, aspirin, or both were the cause of the kidney damage was of little practical importance. The real problem was overuse of these drugs, and this overuse was what made the

pharmaceutical industry a very successful business. He then tried to reason unemotionally. If John had tested only phenacetin, publishing the results would not be unreasonable. Why is the fact that he went further and started to study aspirin and acetaminophen (a substance that phenacetin is converted to in the body) in a similar manner; but the animals died causing such a problem? John is suppressing data which throws a different light on the situation. The reason to do the study is to determine what causes the kidney damage in humans who abuse these headache preparations, Singling out one constituent for study at a time is legitimate, but suppressing significant data on the others is wrong. John told Harry he intended to study the other drugs later, but some mention of the experiment he had already completed is necessary not to mislead. The truth and the whole truth is necessary. You can't do ten experiments and pick the results from three which support your contention while ignoring the other seven. Data may be discarded if one has a legitimate reason such as evidence to suggest faulty technique or sample mix-ups, but the results themselves can't be ignored because the experimenter dislikes them. That would be telling nature what it does, not watching it to find out. He would be having more contact with John Block on the Search Committee, a good chance to observe the man.

It is funny, he thought, how coincidence seem to occur. Three months ago this would have largely been an interesting abstract problem in logic. Now it has a practical and emotional side for me as well. At this time I can't discuss this with Reggie Pate of Rule Pharmaceutical because of Harry's confidence. He was beginning to see how easy it is to develop a conflict of interest.

Jim, at the eating club in Chester with Reggie and Roger Brandon, dined in a separate room where members who desired privacy could eat. As usual, the food was excellent, and Jim was torn between having a cocktail and wanting full control of his persuasive powers. He compromised and drank a glass of ale with his meal. At first the conversation was limited to local Chester politics and Jim having little to contribute thoroughly enjoyed his lunch. Reggie suddenly turned to him and asked, "What's up? You sounded like the cat who swallowed the canary on the phone."

Jim was caught with a full mouth. He chewed and swallowed, looking from Reggie's smiling face to Roger's mildly curious glances. As soon as he was able he blurted "Burnett's syndrome!" Seeing no recognition in their faces, he realized his stupidity in expecting two laymen to understand his gist when few physicians would know the condition by its discoverer's name. By now all food was swallowed and he could speak normally.

"Burnett's syndrome is a medical condition in which many organs, especially the kidneys, are damaged by the excessive intake of calcium. The calcium collects in these organs producing deposits which interfere with normal functioning. The patients suffering from this condition get it by drinking too much milk. They drink several quarts every day for many years; but, to my knowledge, none has sued the dairy.

Reggie nodded as comprehension dawned. "I like it. What do you think, Roger?"

Roger was chewing. Now it was his turn to swallow before speaking. "How common is this condition?" he asked brusquely.

"Not very. I don't know the exact incidence, but it's the idea I'm interested in."

"The fact that patients haven't sued the dairy, assuming none has, isn't much of a precedent upon which to base a case."

"You're missing the point, Mr. Brandon," Jim went on. "I can't imagine a jury holding the dairy responsible for someone with that condition, and dairies don't even put a warning on the carton."

"By comparison, we look good," Reggie chimed in happily.

"I understand what you are getting at, but it isn't very impressive." Roger Brandon was clearly unenthusiastic.

"It seems a good argument to me," added Reggie "It represents a condition brought about by the clear misuse of a product and it points up the absurdity of the situation. I agree with Jim. I still like it."

"But I'm the one who must ultimately decide upon the strategy of our case." Roger was clearly annoyed.

"You don't feel the situations are similar?' asked Jim.

"I didn't say that. I am just not convinced a judge or jury will feel it is relevant to our situation."

"Well I think it is!" Reggie's voice had a clearly authoritative air. "Give it very serious consideration."

On that note, the subject was dropped. Jim left Chester after lunch, mildly deflated, but with Reggie's assurances that Roger would be calling on him for further consultation.

"You sent for me Dr. Green?" Bill Michaelson stood in the doorway of Audrey's laboratory. As usual she sat at her microscope viewing slides. She turned and, recognizing her visitor, rose and invited him to sit at the small work table surrounded by several wooden chairs on one side of the large room. She sat in another and began to sort through some papers and slides which lay on the table.

"Bill, I've gotten together all these data on Runquist so that we can decide how to publish. This whole idea was yours so I feel you ought to write it up and be the senior author. I haven't discussed this with Jim Kulp as yet, but I know him well enough that I'm certain he will agree. He and I would be collaborators."

Bill was flattered and surprised. He had not thought of this eventuality and was at a loss for words Audrey went on, "I personally want to congratulate you and Mrs. Beardsley for the professional manner in which you two handled the whole episode. I was clearly impressed."

"Thank you, Dr. Green. I really appreciate that. I'll tell Donna."

"Please do. Now about a publication: have you had a chance to write anything? I know you have seen all this," she said motioning to the papers on the table.

"I wrote a one page summary of our work and, of course, I wrote the whole study in a complete form on Tommy's chart." Audrey noted a hesitant note in Bill's voice and she waited for him to say something more.

When he didn't, she asked, "Is something troubling you?"

Bill looked uncomfortable. "I don't think we have anything we can publish."

"What do you mean?"

"The study was fine as far as it went, but the results are inconclusive."

"But you and Donna amassed a great deal of data," Audrey insisted. "Surely there is something worth publishing.".

"I honestly don't think so, Dr. Green and believe me I've gone over this in my mind many times."

"It seems such a waste." Audrey sounded disappointed.

"Let me go over my thoughts with you and see if you don't agree." As Audrey said nothing, Bill went on. "The most exciting of the data we have are the blood sugars showing the big dip in the blood sugar curve after alloxan administration and the absence of insulin activity in the tumor and metastasis sample taken post mortem. The trouble is that the way they were taken we can't be sure we got good samples, or enough, and we didn't have any control samples taken before alloxan administration that showed insulin activity. Our data are suggestive at best."

Audrey frowned. "I hate to think of all that suffering and all your work going to waste."

"Believe me, Dr. Green I feel the same way; but when I look at the whole study carefully, I come up with too many holes to want to publish it. If we had other data from some more patients, I wouldn't hesitate to add this to it; but, by itself, I can't see it."

"What does Jim think?"

"Pretty much the same."

Audrey sighed, "Too bad. You all worked so hard. It was clear to Bill that Audrey was unhappy with his decision. "What do you think about the autopsy slides you looked at. Do they help tell us anything?"

"Audrey smiled, recognizing Bill's ploy of placing some responsibility in her area. "Unfortunately, that too is inconclusive. If we could have obtained permission for a legal post mortem, we might have salvaged something. As it was we had a sampling problem. Groping in the dark that way turned out to be unsatisfactory."

"I really would like to publish, but I honestly don't believe we would be adding a thing to the scientific literature," said Bill earnestly.

"I'm impressed by your candor, Bill," Audrey smiled, "and your respect for science. I fear it is a rare individual who questions whether his contribution to the literature is really a contribution. We take it for granted that what we do is important. Our very reputations in science seem to depend upon the number of publications we have amassed. To make the list longer, some fragment one piece of work into several smaller pieces and then publish and republish the same data in several places. Most journals require original data, but few ever check to be sure. I like your style, Bill. Don't change. Don't ever change."

Bill was embarrassed. He had never seen this side of Audrey and he was clearly unused to such attention. He rose to go, assuming his visit was at an end. Realizing her effusive outbreak had embarrassed him, she changed the subject.

"Are you enjoying obstetrics?" she asked.

Bill thought a moment. "It's too soon to say. I think I will. I find it quite similar to surgery except for the area of attention and the dearth of male patients."

"You know, you're right, Bill, I never considered it that way. We do have lots in common with obstetrics and gynecology."

"In some ways, Dr. Green, it's a happier service. The patients leave with something added rather than removed. It's a more pleasant atmosphere in which to work."

"Are you considering specializing?"

"I don't know. I enjoy research, but I'll wait until I've rotated through all the services before I make any decisions."

"That's wise You might even consider surgical pathology. We are always looking for good people."

"Thank you, Dr. Green., I'm complimented."

"You should be." Audrey had now returned to her microscope and Bill realized he was being dismissed.

Tony Lewis corrected his portion of a written examination the Pharmacology Department had given to second year students. In this examination, Tony had several "fill in the blank" questions. He had made no list of answers from which the students could draw; but; instead, relied on the students being able to remember the answers from reading the textbook or from notes taken in his lectures. As he checked the answers in one student's examination, he began laughing. The student was obviously guessing and had made up a chemical substance which did not and could not exist. "Bromine sulfate," read Tony. How could he possibly come up with that imaginary salt of two anions? He marked it wrong and continued to be amused even though appalled at the training in chemistry that medical student must have acquired in college.

Several minutes later, he was startled to find the same absurd answer to the same question on another student's paper. This cannot be a coincidence, he thought.. There isn't any place that answer could have come from but someone's distorted imagination. One of these two must be copying. He then compared other mistakes on these same two papers and was unhappy to find other instances of the same wrong answers. These, at least, were possible answers and by themselves would not have aroused suspicion, but coupled with "Bromine sulfate" they did. Tony took the papers down the hall to Bob Mettlar's office where he shared his discovery with Bob.

"Have any other students given that answer?" Bob inquired.

"I don't know," Tony answered, "I've only gone through a quarter of the tests so far."

"I can't imagine an explanation other than copying," said Bob, "but if you are going to copy, why copy from an idiot?"

Tony chuckled and asked, "What should we do about this, Bob?"

"First, you had better see the rest of the tests to be sure what we are dealing with here. Let the rest of the faculty grading these test know so they can be on the lookout for possible signs of cheating. When the exams are fully graded we will have to prepare a report and turn it over to the student honor society. They administer the honor code."

Tony finished checking the rest of the examinations and could find no definitive evidence of cheating. He passed the exams along to Rodney Barrett who laughed heartily when he saw the first blank containing "Bromine sulfate" but stopped abruptly when shown the second on the other exam.

"Oh no!" he exclaimed, "you know what Jake Bourne said about the honor system, 'the faculty has the honor and the students have the system'. We are not allowed to proctor examinations which suits me just fine. Catching a clever cheater isn't easy besides the students have all been indoctrinated into the honor code. They agree not to give or receive aid during examinations and to turn in anyone they see cheating. And they all sign a statement to that effect when they turn in their papers. The idea of an honor system is a good one. The expectation that they will turn in cheaters is unrealistic. That is squealing and we are taught early in life not to squeal. When the honor system doesn't work, the honest student suffers as his grades are relatively lower and he may lose out on prestigious internships and residencies."

"That may well be; but in this case," Tony explained, "the impetus to cheat was merely to pass the course and stay in school, not to be top of the class."

When the entire examination was graded, no further strong evidence appeared, though other parts of the test tended to corroborate the transfer of information between the authors of the two exams in question. Who stole from whom and who was guilty or innocent of any honor code infringement could not be ascertained.

The students involved were Terry Brown and Randy Branch. Their papers, along with the Pharmacology faculty's assessment of the situation, were turned over to the honor society.

Leonard Stagg, a fourth year medical student almost through with his course of study, was awaiting word as to where he would be going for his internship. His grades, among the best, led him to hope for the prestigious Massachusetts General hospital.

When he complied with Dean Mackenzie's summons he expected to have his answer. He was disappointed to find the subject matter discussed far different from his expectation. In his role as president of the honor society he had, so far, only pleasurable duties. Now he was to be burdened with an unhappy duty: that of convening the society to deal with an accusation of cheating. The Dean told him the story and showed him the absurd answers involved. Dean Mackenzie had also let him know that Terry Brown, one of the students involved, was the son of a classmate who just happened to be on the Board of Trustees of the Massachusetts General Hospital. This bit of news had been so skillfully relayed that it wasn't until Leonard had left the Dean's presence that the possible significance of it hit him. He had never before been "pressured" and he was truly uncertain as to whether he was being so now. Why mention the fact unless it had significance, he reasoned? I may be naive, but I'm not stupid. Still, he wasn't sure.

He called his committee together to discuss the problem. It was made up of two students from each of the four classes. Dr. Alfred Crane of Medicine was the faculty advisor. He did not attend meetings unless requested to do so by the committee, and served in a purely advisory capacity. Whatever the committee decided was passed on to the Dean to implement. No one could remember a time the committee's recommendation had been ignored.

"You can see from these examination papers that there is strong circumstantial evidence of copying. As there is no such chemical as 'bromine sulfate', it is pretty hard to see how two students could have come up with the same wrong answer except by passing information between them. I think we had better have them in for a confrontation. Does anyone see it differently?"

"Who is making the accusation?" a committee member asked.

"The answer was on Dr. Tony Lewis's part of the pharmacology quiz."

"Shouldn't we talk with him about this?" the same student asked.

"A report of the incident was included in the letter I sent telling you of this meeting. Didn't you read it?" Leonard asked.

"Yes, but I would still like to ask him some questions," the student persisted.

"All right. I'll let you all know when we can meet again with all the principals involved. If no one has anything further to add, let's adjourn."

"I hear you've been summoned by the honor society, "Jim Kulp remarked to Tony the next day when they passed in the hall outside of the departmental office.

"Good news travels fast," answered Tony with a wry smile.

"What can they ask you that you haven't already said in your report?"

"Beats me. I can't imagine. I can't shed any light on which, if either, of those boys is guilty."

"What do you mean, 'if either'?"

"There could be another explanation, Jim."

"Like what, for instance?"

"There you have me. I can't honestly conceive of one."

"Tony, you know the maxim in medicine that you never invoke a complicated explanation when a simple one will do."

"I know, I know but the evidence you must admit is circumstantial."

"Hell, Tony, I don't care what they do. I just don't like them badgering you. All you did was bring it to their attention."

"No one's badgering me."

"Not yet maybe, but I bet they grill you, and furthermore I'll lay you odds no one gets punished. Want to bet?"

"No thanks, Jim."

That afternoon Dr. Lewis met with the students. He was truly surprised by the accuracy of Jim's predictions. The students were polite but he had the feeling he was on trial, not the students. Tony was an exceptionally even tempered person and kept himself under good control. He kept telling himself the students were merely trying to get to the bottom of the strange answers and were not hostile to him as they appeared. He pointed out to them he was not trying to undermine the honor code and believed in it himself, though he was aware there were many on the faculty who didn't. At one point, he asked in complete exasperation, "What would you have done in my place: ignored the strange coincidence?"

No one answered. The questioners then took a new tack.

"Suppose," Leonard Stagg asked "these two students study together, as they claim they do, couldn't that answer have mistakenly gotten into one of their class notes and been copied by the other when studying and then reproduced on the test? In essence, no infringement of the honor code had to occur."

"That's certainly possible," Tony admitted.

"You don't feel that is likely?" another student asked in a slightly sneering fashion.

"That is a judgment your committee must make. My feelings are immaterial," Tony answered without rancor.

"Dr. Lewis," another student asked, "can you think of anything you might have told the students which even remotely sounds like 'bromine sulfate'?"

"No, I can't."

"Is there anything in their text?"

"I don't understand your question," said Tony.

"Is there anything in their textbooks that sounds like..." The student, realizing that textbooks don't make sounds blushed as he comprehended the ridiculousness of his question.

Tony answered, "I racked my brain to come up with an explanation other than a possible infringement of the honor code before the report was turned over to you. I am truly sorry to say I was unable to do so."

As there were no further questions, Leonard thanked Tony for appearing before them and being so patient. After Tony left the room, the discussion centered on possible ways in which the odd answer could have appeared other than outright stupidity and cheating. No remotely reasonable explanation was forthcoming. A few students reverted to anger with Tony Lewis for dumping the problem in their laps. Others rejected that view and felt the students involved ought to be punished; but which one? The meeting was adjourned.

"So that's where it stands." Leonard Stagg was in Al Crane's office and had filled him in on the details of the meeting and problem. "Dr. Crane, I'm stumped. I really do not know what to do. The committee has reached no consensus. This is our first experience in this sort of situation. Can you help us?"

Al Crane had listened carefully during the entire recital. His high brow wrinkled in intense concentration. The furrows smoothed and a smile appeared on his face. He leapt from his chair and crossed the room to a bookshelf against the opposite wall. He scanned the shelves and soon pulled a thick reference book and brought it back to his desk where he turned the pages rapidly, stopped suddenly and laughingly shouted, "Eureka!" while pointing to a place on the page for Leonard, who thought he'd gone mad, to see.

When the committee later made known its findings to the Dean, it completely exonerated the students who misheard Dr. Lewis in his lecture concerning "bromine cyanide." The explanation wasn't too farfetched under the circumstances and it did serve to get everyone off the hook.

Bob Mettlar put things in perspective when he observed, "With all its faults the honor system relieves us of having to match wits with dishonest students. Those who are determined to cheat will outsmart me. A majority of our students are honest and conscientious. The few who are not should be removed by their peers.

When Jim Kulp next saw Tony Lewis, Tony admitted Jim's predictions had been correct. Jim asked him what he thought of the committee's explanation of confusing "bromine sulfate" and "bromine cyanide". Tony shrugged. "It may sound logical except I have always called that substance 'cyanogen bromide'. I was not aware of that other name."

Terry Brown, feeling under a cloud of suspicion was unhappy. Guilty of stupidity for filling blanks at the last moments of a test with wild guesses in the hopes of gaining a few more points, but that was all. He was not dishonest. He had not seen anyone copying from his paper and, therefore, had not violated the honor code.

Randy Branch was either psychic or lying. It did seem too much to ask of coincidence. He told all he knew to the committee but did not feel he was being believed. He did not know what Randy had told them. They had not spoken since the accusation surfaced.

The committee's recommendation came, at first, as a relief; but as he thought more and more about it, the unhappier he became. It gave everyone an "out" but no satisfaction. He suspected no one believed that explanation. He knew it was wrong. Damn it, he thought. Why do I feel so uncomfortable? I've done nothing wrong. Compared to Randy my grades are worse and I have to work harder for them than he seems to. If he copied from my paper, especially that dumb answer, he mustn't be too bright. All his grades may be phony. I'll watch him more closely from now on.

Randy came from a long line of Branches who were doctors. He knew he, too, would be a doctor, for as far back as he could remember. He didn't object, neither was he enthusiastic. He would be another doctor as were his father, mother, sisters and brothers, all older. They lived in a sizable city to the West and most practiced there though a few had managed to leave the state. As the youngest of the present Branch crop, he had received lots of attention, and the expectations for him were high. In high school he had been tutored by older, smarter siblings, and he managed to do well. He was not stupid and did better with one to one tutoring. Left to his own devices, he was not driven and found that applying himself to subjects in which he wasn't interested impossible. As a result his grades would suffer. When this would happen his family's disappointment dismayed him. Had he told them he would prefer some other field than medicine they would have supported him without truly understanding. They were, after, all kindly sympathetic people and these attributes made them good clinicians. They were a loving family and their obvious wishes for him became coercive, much more so than had they been demands. Randy had never seriously considered treading some other pathway but took the simple expedient of helping poor grades along by copying from crib notes, other student or any available source that worked for him. He would rationalize his transgressions by dutifully learning the material he had cribbed after the examination. He never tried for top grades, just enough to keep him pointed towards his family's goal for him.

In medical school the situation grew worse. All courses were scientific, so he hadn't the benefit of any which truly stimulated him. He resorted more and more to dishonest means of passing, and he was having more and more trouble rationalizing his behavior. He became morose, short tempered and his relationship with those around him suffered. He was definitely considered an oddball by his fellow students. His few friendly relationships evaporated, and by his second year he was truly miserable. His family, whose contacts with him were limited to his few and brief vacations, saw him at his best which, though none too good, was ascribed by them to the rigors and demands of second year medical school. They tried to encourage him by describing the fun and excitement of the clinical years and patient care and were unworried, for that important diagnostic sign, his grades, were satisfactory.

The current fiasco, copying asinine answers from Terry Brown, brought home the truth. The game he was playing could not continue. It was almost as if he wanted to be caught and end the charade at any cost. Still he could imagine the hurt in the eyes of his parents were he to be expelled for cheating. He would be unable to face that. The committee had exonerated them. What a laugh If only he could have been honest with them, but there was no way. I suppose they'll be watching me now, he thought, and Terry too, poor guy, not overly bright, but honest. My stupidity is beginning to hurt others and they don't deserve that. Oh God what can I do? His eyes filled with tears as the misery and loneliness of his present life closed in on him. It was noon, and he was due at a pharmacology lab in one hour. He went into the bathroom to wash his face and try to erase the redness around his eyes. At the washbowl another wave of sorrow struck him. He stood hunched over sobbing. He straightened up and opened the medicine cabinet behind the sink avoiding his reflection in the mirror. Through his tears he saw his solution, a bottle of phenobarbital capsules. "I didn't want to go to laboratory this afternoon anyway," he said aloud to no one in particular, "not tomorrow nor the next day." He considered writing a note, but what could he say. They would figure it out. Again he burst into tears. He sat on his bed and began to swallow pills which he washed down with water. By the time they were all gone, he was getting drowsy so he slipped out of his clothes and climbed between the sheets feeling better than he had for ages.

Terry looked for Randy in the laboratory that afternoon. He was determined to try to clear himself and he felt Randy was the key. He had considered going to Dr. Lewis and proclaiming his innocence, but what would that accomplish? He had tried to get information on the kind of person Randy was, but he was unsuccessful. No one seemed to know much about him. He kept to himself, he didn't have friends, male or female, and the word "odd" kept appearing in the conversations Terry had. No one had anything good or bad to say about him and that in itself was unusual. Terry wanted to see his grades and transcripts hoping for some clue, but he could not determine how to do this. He had finally decided to confront him directly. Hell he owes me an answer, he thought. It was my paper he copied from. His disappointment in not finding him in the student laboratory session was great since he had finally mustered the courage to confront him and he was impatient to do so. Something else about Randy's unusual absence was beginning to disturb him.

He went to Dr. Lewis and asked for permission to go and find Randy. Tony took the time to discuss his unusual request with him once he realized how upset Terry was. They found a place in the student laboratory away from the others and must have talked for forty minutes. No one knew where Randy lived so it was some time before they were able to locate his residence and phone number from the Dean's office files. The phone was busy and continued to be so for over the twenty minutes Terry dialed it from Tony's office. At least I know where he is, Terry thought. I'll go and confront him there. Tony encouraged him to go and find Randy realizing he wouldn't learn anything in the laboratory in his present agitated state.

When he finally found the room in which Randy lived, it was almost three-thirty in the afternoon. The door was locked and he could hear no sounds when he placed his ear to the door. He found the landlady and borrowed her phone to call. The busy signal suggested the phone was off the hook.

Seeing Terry's concern she asked, "Is something wrong?"

"I don't know," he responded. "Do you have a key to his room?"

The landlady gave him a pass key and he bounded up the stairs and found Randy's near-lifeless body in the bed. He tried vainly to arouse him and placed his ear against his chest listening for a heartbeat being unable to feel any pulses. He thought he could hear a beat but was unsure when he felt a slight movement of the chest wall as Randy took one of his infrequent breaths.

"He's alive!" Terry shouted to the landlady who had worked up the courage to follow him into Randy's room. Terry leapt from the bed, hung up Randy's phone and dialed the operator for an emergency. He was connected eventually with the emergency room at Wilder General Hospital. He told the nurse on the other end of the line all she needed, and within a few minutes Randy's comatose body was on its way to Wilder. A mask was strapped to his face and oxygen was forced into his lungs periodically by a medical attendant. Terry located the empty bottle of phenobarbital and sent it along with them. He returned to the pharmacology student laboratory by four-fifteen, and one look at his face told Dr. Lewis something was seriously amiss.

"I sensed something wasn't right when he didn't show for lab." said Terry. "It's as though I had a second sense."

"Thank God you did," was all that Tony could think to say.

In the emergency room Randy's condition was assessed. His respirations were so infrequent and his reflexes so depressed that a tracheal tube was threaded through his mouth into his windpipe where a balloon in the tube's outer wall was inflated to seal it to the trachea. He was placed on a positive pressure respirator which breathed for him. A tentative diagnosis of phenobarbital poisoning was made and blood samples sent to the clinical chemistry laboratory to confirm the diagnosis and to try and estimate how much drug had been taken. Stomach tubing and washing were discussed and dispensed with as the depth of coma and the estimates of time since drug ingestion suggested, to those handling the case, they would not be fruitful. Intravenous solutions were started in Randy's veins for future therapy and immediate support for his falling blood pressure.

The resident in charge of the emergency room was Durward Jenkens and he had had a fair amount of experience treating drug overdoses. A case of pure phenobarbital poisoning without numerous other drugs thrown in was in some ways a luxury and the history given in this case, plus what he was seeing, strongly suggested that diagnosis. After several hours, Randy's condition did not improve. If anything, it worsened. Reflexes which were initially markedly depressed were now completely absent. His blood pressure was requiring more and more drugs to maintain it at a safe level. Randy seemed to be worsening. Durward called in John Block, who on hearing the patient was a second year medical student, came to the emergency room to manage the case himself. The laboratory reported highly dangerous levels of phenobarbital on the initial blood samples obtained and higher levels in subsequent samples. On hearing this John Block immediately instituted bicarbonate infusions to hasten the excretion of the drug through the kidneys. He was limited in the degree to which he could institute this particular therapy by fears of overloading Randy's cardiovascular system and producing heart failure. Though Randy was young and strong, phenobarbital in very high doses is depressant to heart muscle. Peter Markley looked in on Randy and suggested this case might be one which could benefit from dialysis as a means of hastening drug removal. John Block considered this suggestion carefully but wanted to await further blood levels before making up his mind. When the six o'clock levels came in even higher than the earlier ones, he agreed with Peter. He was also critical of the residents decision not to wash out the stomach. Despite good supportive therapy and the alkaline diuresis, something more was needed. He sent for Linda Koster. It was now eight in the evening and the Doctors Branch had arrived from thee Western part of the state. They were both pale and quiet and clearly shaken. The fact that they had not known their son was so unhappy upset them most of all. As professionals, they knew something immediate had to be done, and were thankful the accident had occurred here at Wilder where the likes of John Block could care for their son They agreed to the use of dialysis if John wanted to use it and permission was granted.

By nine o'clock, the catheters were placed in the blood stream and the dialysis was begun. It was continued until five the next morning at which time all signs and symptoms of phenobarbital overdose were clearly improving. Linda and the others who had remained by the bedside were feeling the strain of the long night. The fact that they were dealing with a young patient and a medical student contributed to that strain. As is often the case in such circumstances, rumors as to the source of the patient's troubles were rampant, but the most common rumor was near the truth. The sight of the distraught parents, both doctors, was a strong impetus to all to want to save this patient, and at this point they felt they had.

Randy slept for another twenty-four hours but without the aid of dialysis, a respirator or blood pressure raising infusions. By the third day, Randy could converse with his parents, though no intelligent discussions could take place.

Dean Mackenzie had followed the case closely from its inception and had spent time discussing Randy with Terry Brown, Tony Lewis, and Randy's parents. He rightly deduced Randy should not be in Medicine unless he, Randy, wanted to be and he now suspected he didn't. He assigned Phil Schuyler, a psychiatrist with an excellent record with students, to get to the bottom of the matter as soon as Randy's condition would allow, and Phil began by interviewing the Doctors Branch who tried to be as helpful as possible and were clearly concerned.

Tony Lewis summarized the situation. "What started as an error on a pharmacology quiz grew to a near tragedy and has ended with a student leaving medical school for a more suitable life's work. In the process, a clinical report showing dialysis is capable of removing considerable amounts of phenobarbital from a human's blood stream was born. One student's reputation was completely cleared while another's relationship with loving parents has been markedly improved. Some of the honor society members are chagrined while others are saying 'I told you so'."

Leonard Stagg who was at first full of admiration for Alfred Crane, was now not so sure. Dr. Crane still thought he had come up with a great solution at the time. "If you are going to make it in medical school administration, you've got to learn to lie a little," he chuckled to himself.

SPRING

Spring came to Wilder after a long winter. An annual sign of spring was the student-faculty picnic in which the entire medical school assembled for beer, athletics and merriment. The morning of the picnic a special meeting of the Search Committee had been called.

"We have now been visited by three candidates," John Block summarized.

"Two of these have already declined further consideration. This leaves only Sidney Amstel to be considered for the position from ninety prospective candidates we have explored. Dean Mackenzie wants us to speed up the proceedings as much as we can. That is why I called this meeting. What are your feelings about Dr. Amstel?" he asked.

"I was impressed with him," Professor Root allowed in his usual grave and ponderous manner, "I think he would make a splendid chairman. He seems to have administrative ability, and he certainly impressed Frank Mackenzie on his recent visit."

"He did that all right," added Dick Shane. "He boned up on his history of medicine in this state and knew exactly how to win Frank over. I have to admire his skill."

"I thought he was a personable young man, suave, urbane perhaps too much so for this rural school," said Professor Evans, the oldest member of the committee. "I wonder what he sees in us?"

"Though Dr. Amstel is the only outside candidate left, we haven't written off all insiders, have we?" interrupted Jim Kulp.

"Whom do you have in mind?" asked John Block.

"Rodney Barret," answered Jim.

"All right, why don't we consider him right now. You all have Dr. Barret's resume and Dr. Amstel's. Let's compare the two.

Some minutes were spent discussing the relative merits of the two candidates. Dr. Barret was well known to all the members of the committee, while Dr. Amstel was only an acquaintance of Jim Kulp's. Surprisingly, to Jim, Dr. Barret's proximity did not seem to be a positive influence on most of the committee.

Jim, though acquainted with Amstel and having nothing against him, clearly preferred Rodney Barret. He felt his preference for Barret was conceived in unselfish reasoning. He knew Rodney was sought after by other schools and would probably soon leave Wilder if he were not selected chairman. That would be, he thought, a serious loss for the department and the school. He was also aware of Rodney's compulsive drive having lost research space to him. At the time that had occurred, he was disappointed but had to admit that Rodney had made better use of the space than he would have. Rodney was clearly destined for accomplishment in his field of research. Sidney Amstel, on the other hand had not distinguished himself as a researcher.

Jim was friendly with Sidney, had acted as his host on his visit to Wilder, and would, he thought, be able to exert more personal influence on him than would the other department members were he chosen head. He dismissed that selfish consideration from his deliberations. In essence, he felt Rodney Barret clearly the better man for the position and would be disappointed if the committee chose Amstel.

Dick Shane had turned to the pages of both resumes which contained the candidates' publications. Without looking up he observed, "Dr. Amstel has twenty published paper and Dr. Barret has only sixteen." For a moment there was silence.

In a rather incredulous voice Jim Kulp inquired "If you are really serious about that comparison, Dick, don't you think we ought to read the papers?"

"That's not necessary, Dr. Kulp. I note they are all in reputable journals," the surgeon countered. As the only reply that came to Jim's mind was obscene, he refrained from making one.

"Are there any other candidates we should consider?" John Block asked. No one spoke. "Gentlemen, we have before us two candidates for the possible chairmanship of the Pharmacology Department. Though our recommendation is not final, in that the candidate must be acceptable to the Executive Committee made up of all the department heads, we will in all probability make the choice. Is there any more discussion on the two before us?" John asked.

Jim Kulp was astonished at the rapidity with which things were moving. It was true that it had taken eight months to arrive at their present position, but he had imagined that there would be much more discussion concerning the relative merits of Amstel and Barret. He had expected Professor Evans to advocate Rodney

Barret and was puzzled by his silence. Barret and Evans had worked in the same field and even published together. He thought Evans held Barret in high esteem. None of the committee members said a word. Kulp wanted to say something, to get some discussion going; but he was the youngest, least experienced member of the committee and, from the impassive expressions on the faces of the others, felt his words would be resented and might even hurt Rodney's chances.

"Shall we simply have a show of hands?" John Block asked. Following a few nods, he went on, "those in favor of Dr. Amstel, please signify your desire." Four hands were raised. "Those in favor of Rodney Barret." A lone hand was raised.

"I didn't need to vote, but just so there will be no misunderstanding," John Block said while glaring at Jim, "I would have voted for Dr. Amstel. It appears we favor Dr. Amstel. If Frank Mackenzie concurs we'll ask him back for a second visit. As you know, a second visit is tantamount to an offer; in fact, a serious offer can be made at that time. Anything more?"

As no one was responding to his question, Jim asked, "What about the Executive Committee?"

"If Frank wants him, that will be a rubber stamp. Meeting adjourned. See you at the picnic."

Jim left the meeting without speaking to anyone. He sensed some sort of conspiracy and could not believe that a choice could be made with so little discussion. While true that eight months had passed, the time had been spent sorting out the unwanted and being unwanted by most of the remainder. The few finalists had visited and two of the three had eliminated themselves from consideration. The process had left two candidates whose importance had grown if only by their willingness to take on the task. To dismiss one of them after but a few minutes of superficial deliberation seemed irresponsible to Jim. Something of which he was not aware must have transpired. In a bewildered state of mind he drove home to pick up Janet and the children for the picnic.

He looked forward to the student-faculty picnic. It signaled the end of the course with its heavy teaching load. Though he enjoyed teaching, the time required, particularly during the winter quarter, was great and lessened the time he could spend on his greatest love, research. Then too, by the end of the course he had gotten to know the medical students in his classes reasonably well and he enjoyed the easy fellowship a few beers and a softball game inevitably produced. The presence of other faculty and their families mingling with the students and their families gave a picture of one big happy medical family which Jim thoroughly enjoyed. He wasn't sure he would this year.

He had an uncomfortable feeling, akin to guilt, which had been with him for some time and had been brought to the forefront of his mind during the morning meeting. He suddenly recognized its origin. Though he was familiar with Rodney's research work from their close association, he had never known much of Sidney Amstel's. As he tried to point out in the meeting, he could not imagine seriously considering a candidate to head a scientific department without knowing his scientific abilities. In most cases this meant reading some of the candidate's published work. He had not done so. He rationalized this mistake by assuming the committee would choose Rodney Barret. The reality of what had happened this morning was beginning to penetrate his mind full force. He wanted to tell someone; to talk it over with the departmental members but the meetings, he had been informed, were to be conducted in secrecy and the deliberations were not to be discussed outside of the committee. He had obeyed this stricture although he suspected others of ignoring it. Certain information which had been relayed to him from the other members of his department could have arisen only in the committee meetings.

The weather was perfect for the picnic. The athletic events stimulated appetites and the hot sauce on the barbecue created thirst which the barrels of draft beer helped to slake. By mid-afternoon the party was in full swing and Jim was beginning to relax and enjoy the harmonious feeling he had been afraid he would miss.

For a moment he was seen sitting by himself and Rodney rushed to his side.

"Is it true you're bringing Dr. Amstel down for a second visit?" he asked brusquely.

Jim surprised by the question and the unfriendly manner in which it was asked; hesitated, not knowing how to answer.

"Have you read any of his publications?" Rodney continued in the same unfriendly manner.

Jim shook his head to indicate he had not.

"You damn well better before you bring him here!" Rodney exploded before turning his back and stalking off.

Jim and Rodney were good friends and this hostile encounter startled Jim. He wondered if Rodney was drunk, but nothing in his walk suggested inebriation. His next reactions were anger and disappointment; anger at someone on the committee who was leaking privileged information, disappointment with Rodney who was displaying "sour grapes".

As he calmed down, he seriously considered Rodney's admonition and knew that he must read Amstel's published works as soon as possible. He arranged for his family to return from the picnic with neighbors and proceeded to the medical library. He chose the last six publications listed in the Index Medicus under the name of Sidney B. Amstel and was fortunate to find four of these in bound journals on the shelves. He checked them out and proceeded to his office to read.

Amstel's field of research differed from his own and he was prepared for a long session of intense study which the beer he had ingested might hinder. He was unprepared for what he found. Within one hour he understood Rodney's wrath. The papers were amazing. He could not imagine how they had been able to pass an editor's scrutiny. They were filled with minor errors, slipped decimal points and simple mathematical mistakes. In addition, they were poorly constructed. Jim was reminded of term papers he had written in college for courses he had to take which didn't interest him and were left to the last minute before they were due. Dr. Amstels papers were far from the quality to be acceptable for a scientific department head.

Jim, concerned that the Search Committee was about to make a horrendous mistake, was certain his motives in bringing these papers to their attention would be suspect. He wanted corroboration; but he was concerned about the executive session policy.

Someone on the committee must be guilty of imparting their deliberations. He had not been. Why should he feel guilty about what he was planning to do. His mood elevated and his concerns subsided. He was beginning to feel that even as the junior member of the committee, working in what to him was an unfamiliar area, campus politics, he was going to make a real contribution.

"What is so important that you are getting me out early on a Sunday morning?" Tony Lewis asked with a friendly handshake as he crossed the threshold of the Kulp residence and greeted his host shortly after eight, the day following the picnic.

"Believe it or not, you're the last one here," answered Jim leading Tony into his living room where Bob Mettlar and Professor Mary White, head of the Biochemistry department were having coffee.

After greetings were exchanged, Jim thanked the three of his visitors for joining him on such short notice with no apparent explanation.

"As you are all aware, I am on the Search Committee to choose a head for Pharmacology. The committee has met supposedly in executive sessions; but someone, not me until now, has been reporting our deliberations outside the committee. Who or how this information is leaked isn't important except to justify my own present behavior.

"The committee has decided to recommend Sidney Amstel's name to the Dean. They, to my knowledge, have never read his published work. I hadn't either, I'm ashamed to say until yesterday. Somehow Rodney Barret learned of the committee's recommendation within hours of our making it. He demanded I read Amstel's papers. I did. I want you to read them now. I have made copies for all of you. I included Professor White in this exercise because her reputation as a scientist and lack of affiliation with our department will give more weight to any opinions she may express in the future. I know this is an odd request, but please read these papers. If you wish, I'll keep your reactions to myself. If you react as I suspect you will, I will go to the committee today before we invite Amstel for a second visit. I want your judgment on these papers to be sure my own is not faulty."

Though it was clear none of the three was happy with the early Sunday morning study assignment, they grudgingly began to read. Jim kept the coffee flowing. There was silence marred only by the occasional rustling of paper and the sounds of china coffee cups striking their saucers. As time wore on, Jim was aware of the gamut of emotions growing within him. Not since his final oral Ph.D. examinations had he been so nervous. He wondered whether his friendship and respect for Rodney Barret had poisoned his analytical abilities.

Mary White was the first to break the silence. "I'm ashamed to say some of these papers were published in biochemical journals, not the prestigious ones at any rate. I'm at a loss to know how these got through."

There followed a discussion of journals, publications and the burgeoning scientific literature which resulted from the unintelligent adherence of a majority of scientific institutions to the "publish or perish" concept. An investigator was largely judged by the number of publications authored rather than their contents. This unhappy fact hurt science by filling its literature with garbage and by converting teachers of budding scientists into garbage collectors. The government fostered this trend by enticing more garbage collectors into the field based on the faulty premise that money can always hasten the unlocking of nature's secrets. Though true to a small extent, too much support hurts medical science by attracting medical research entrepreneurs whose chief motivation is the building of medical empires. Many of these empires produce results of questionable value and hurt the quality of teaching and patient care.

Ordinarily Jim would have welcomed such a discussion. He hoped for a more specific critique of the papers and finally interrupted to say so. There followed a prolonged discussion pointing out errors such as he had already noted and even some he had not. Among the latter were two of extreme importance. One was the use of an extraction solvent to remove a particular substance the author wished to measure, from a tissue in which he was to measure it. The problem was that the solvent was known, by Mary White at least, to destroy the substance he wished to measure. While no one is expected to know everything, this particular fact would have been evident had he designed his experiments to include the proper controls on his method of quantification. He could then have substituted the proper solvent.

The second problem they uncovered was of a more serious nature and could be noted only by comparing data from one of Amstel's publications with another. One paper described an experiment done with male mice; another an experiment with females. The control data given for these two separate papers were quantitatively the same. There was no reasonable explanation as to how this could be a simple mistake and, coupled with the myriad of minor errors and generally poor quality of the papers, raised the specter of dishonesty in all their minds, though this aspect was never openly discussed.

Jim now had the support for his judgments of the papers from three eminent and experienced scientists whose objectivity he respected. Knowing that these three had seldom agreed so readily on any other matter further reinforced his feelings. His guests departed and he called John Block at his home and asked if he might come and talk with him. A time was agreed upon for that afternoon.

Prior to the Search Committee, he had spent a little time with John Block getting some advice on analytical methods they both used in their respective researches. Their relationship in the past had always been a cordial one, that of a young investigator and a seasoned veteran. Jim's faith in John's objectivity had been seriously shaken by the phenacetin experiment John and Harry Tatum had done, but he felt the best way to proceed was through the chairman of the Search Committee. Jim was certain that once Amstel's published work was made known to John he would recognize that Amstel was not an acceptable choice. Once that had occurred John could easily convince the other members of the Search Committee.

John welcomed him warmly and listened to his story in silence. Jim did not tell him of his meeting earlier in the day with Mettlar, Lewis and White. When he finished, John asked him to leave Amstel's publications with him so that he could study them. He promised to call Jim in a few hours. Jim left feeling John would make a formidable opponent at a poker table as he had no idea how his presentation had been received. He returned home to await John's summons.

Not far away in her living room sat Marie Barret surrounded by her loved ones all except Rodney. She was an intensely religious Catholic and Sunday afternoon after church had been her happiest time of the week. Rodney had made a special effort not to work on Sunday and this was her "taking-stock-and-planning" day in her previously well ordered life. Now there were complications. She was dialyzed on Monday, Wednesday and Friday; and Sunday fell on her longest inter-dialytic period. This meant that on Sunday her blood and tissues were filled with the highest levels of products of her bodily metabolism which normally are rapidly excreted by normally functioning kidneys. Though Sunday was an extra holiday from that "infernal machine", it was also the day she tended to feel the worst. Her taking stock and planning was no longer enjoyable as she had difficulty seeing very far into the future and was only just beginning to come to terms with her condition. From what she was learning of end stage renal disease, it seemed a slow down hill course with little respite to look to unless one considered a possible transplant operation. Then, too, she was having difficulty getting

Rodney to face these troubles with her. For a short while he had become more interested in her plight and more supportive. Slowly, however, they seemed to be growing apart, and yesterday Rodney appeared hostile. Something had happened and Rodney had left the picnic without telling her. She had seen him talking briefly with Jim Kulp and then later she had seen him with Linda Koster. When it came time to leave the picnic, he was nowhere to be found so she rounded up the children and drove home without him. Occasionally at these picnics, Rodney would drink too much beer and be brought home by a friend. Marie was thus not overly worried and dozed off expecting to awaken when Rodney returned. Now it was Sunday and he still hadn't. She had gone to church without him and feeling he was away by his own volition, did not make any inquiries. The children being used to Daddy's long work hours did not question his absence.

In still another part of town, Rodney Barret lay flat on his back with his eyes closed. His head ached with an intensity he recognized and swore never to self-impose again. He opened his eyes and instantly remembered that alcohol was not the only complication. He was in a strange bedroom, in a strange bed and was not alone. Though the blinds were drawn, he could see the outline of his bed mate, though his mind was rapidly recalling events that made it unnecessary for him to look closer for purposes of identification. Rodney had never before been unfaithful to his wife, but yesterday he had been so with a vengeance. It was not that he didn't love Marie. He did; but he was used to an active sex life, and

Marie's illness had changed that. The sudden realization that he was not to be offered the departmental chairmanship and that it might go to a scientific inferior outsider had shocked and infuriated him. He had blasted Jim Kulp at the picnic and being ashamed had relied on beer to improve his mood. He had run into Linda, and feeling the need for a stronger drink and not trusting his ability to drive, he had invited her to chauffeur him home for some whiskey. She changed his plan and they went to her apartment which was adequately supplied. One thing led to another and now it was Sunday. He could not recall clearly making love to her, but a local tenderness told him he had been up to a lot of something, and his lack of depression suggested that he had enjoyed himself. He couldn't understand why he wasn't feeling remorse and shame, but he wasn't. Linda stirred. Strange odors began to enter his consciousness at once repelling and enticing him. Despite the local tenderness, he was thinking how good it would be to have Linda now that he was sober enough to sense the event. He might as well sin a lot as a little. He reached out to her and she responded.

The call came and Jim Kulp hastened to John Block's. When he turned into the Block driveway, he saw Dick Shane entering the house. He was greeted by John and Dick. The latter appeared nervous and was less friendly toward him than Jim could remember during their acquaintance.

"What's all this nonsense about Amstel's scientific incompetence?" Dick demanded as soon as the three were settled in the Block living room.

"I never said he was scientifically incompetent. I showed John some serious flaws in his papers," replied Jim annoyed and wondering why Dick Shane was here at this point.

"John and I have read these papers, and we don't think they're bad."

Jim was stunned. He knew the papers had been read by several capable people.

"Is that so, John? You don't feel the work is poor?" Jim asked looking carefully at John who answered without hesitation.

"They aren't the most important papers written, but neither are they as bad as you seem to think."

"You mean you still want Amstel to head Pharmacology after reading these?"

"You're damned right!" Shane forcefully exclaimed. "To give you the benefit of any doubt, we called Drs. Braun and Sidney and they both vouch for Amstel's scientific competence."

Jim was incredulous. Why didn't you call his Mother, he wondered. Braun and Sidney were co-authors on many of Amstel's papers. "That's not a very impartial source of information," he stated quietly.

"Are you questioning the scientific competence of men of their stature?" Shane asked.

Jim stifled a strong urge to scream "Yes" and realized he was not making any impression on Shane and Block, and he desperately wanted them to see his side. He restrained his natural impulse to suggest that the calling of Amstel's associates was a serious breach of the Search Committee's stated policies. He did not know what their conversation had entailed but he could not imagine receiving a query concerning an acquaintances scientific abilities from a medical school in the market for a department head, and on a Sunday, without raising serious and embarrassing questions. These men might be older and more experienced than he, but they were behaving stupidly. He decided to play what he considered his trump card.

"There is one aspect of these papers that is seriously perplexing," Jim began while picking up two of the copied papers. "In this study done with male mice and in this one done with female mice, the control data are the same."

John carefully compared the papers. After a pause he asked. "Are you calling Amstel a liar?"

"No, John, I'm saying the control data come from the same mice in those two papers."

"Are you calling Amstel a liar?" John persisted.

"No! But those data are the same."

"Then you are calling him a liar."

"If lying is the only explanation you can think of, then you are calling him a liar, but I'm not." Jim insisted.

"How do you know the control data from those two papers are the same?" John changed his tack.

"Because quantitative biological experimental data of that complexity do not repeat themselves exactly. You know that as well as I do, John."

"Have you ever done fractionation experiments like those?" John asked.

"No I haven't"

"Then how do you know they won't repeat that precisely?"

"John! No biological experiments give that sort of precision. Hell, duplicate determinations are seldom that reproducible!"

"Well, if you have never done such experiments, maybe Amstel is just a better experimenter than you are," John countered.

Jim could feel this discussion degenerating.

"I'm sure he is, John, but no one is this good," Jim said pointing to the two papers Dick Shane was studying intensely.

"These aren't the same, look here." Dick pointed to two tables of data. "In the beta fraction in one study you find 32.7 percent and in the other 17.3 percent," he said with glee.

Without taking his eyes off John Block's face, Jim quietly replied, "The 17.3 is the beta one fraction. If you add the beta two and beta three fractions to it you come out with 32.7 percent. In one of the papers he subfactionated the beta fraction."

Dick added the subfractions. Getting the expected result, his face got red and he slammed his pencil down on the table where he sat.

"Goddamn nit picker and boy scout," he hissed between clenched teeth.

"John, I don't seem to be doing a very good job convincing you that these papers are unacceptable for a department head in this school. This work is not in my field. Perhaps someone expert in this field should go over these papers point by point with the entire committee."

"Whom do you have in mind?"

"Of all the people at Wilder, I would say Rodney Barret is the most knowledgeable in this field."

"He is certainly not unbiased in this situation," Dick Shane sputtered..

"I'll grant you that," Jim agreed, "but he would be acting as a guide, not a judge. If he can't point out poor research, it really doesn't matter that…"

John interrupted. "Did Barret point out these flaws to you?"

"Rodney insisted I read Amstel's papers before we invited him for a second visit and I did. That's my reason for haste. I wanted to apprise you of the situation before you invited him a second time.

"How did Barret know we were considering a second visit?" John asked in an accusatory manner.

"I don't know, John, but he knew by the time I talked with him at the picnic. Someone isn't complying with the executive session order. You haven't invited Amstel down yet, have you?"

John Block ignored the question and was silent for a moment before he spoke.

"Perhaps we should have Barret present these papers to the entire committee. I'll call such a meeting for as soon as possible this week."

It was apparent to Jim that John clearly wanted him to leave. He excused himself and left the two men's presence. No sooner had he gone than John turned to the surgeon.

"Well how did your visit with the Dean go?"

Dick winced. "Not well. He was furious. He said we had better get Amstel down here and ensconced damned soon."

"Doesn't he realize we have a problem?"

"Apparently not," Shane answered. What he did not tell John Block, and what he was trying to put out of his mind, was one of his answers to the Dean's questions. When he told Frank Mackenzie that some question concerning Amstel's published papers had arisen, the Dean had angrily inquired, "You've read the papers, haven't you?" At that point Shane had not the courage to be truthful.

"As some of you already know, Rodney has raised serious questions about Sidney Amstel's published papers. What you may not know is that the Committee is seriously considering bringing Amstel down for a second visit." Jim was talking to the full faculty of the Department of Pharmacology in the departmental library and meeting room. This was the first time all six faculty members had met to discuss the selection of their new head. Jim went on. "As a member of the Search Committee, I am supposed to keep the committee's deliberations secret. I wanted to reassure all of you that things were progressing well and to minimize the uncertainty associated with the selection of a new head. Lately, I have reason to believe others on the Search Committee are not following the imposed executive session rule.. The basis of the rumors you have asked me about could have their origins only in our committee's sessions. I will, therefore, no longer remain silent if I perceive giving you 'privileged' information will serve a useful and calming purpose. Feel free to ask about anything that may be troubling you."

"What questions have Amstel's publications raised?" one of the junior departmental members asked.

"Rodney, since you raised the questions, would you care to answer?" Jim replied.

"Dr. Amstel works in a field closely related to my own. His papers were never very significant and until now I never read them. The title and summary were enough to tell me they were not of interest to me. When I heard he might be seriously considered as the new head, I did read some of them. I found he was not just an undistinguished worker, he was an extremely poor investigator. I would be embarrassed to be part of a department of which he was head." Complete silence followed Rodney's statement.

Jim broke the silence. "Before I read Amstel's stuff, I would have been shocked and suspicious of Rodney for the remarks such as he has just made. Now that is no longer the case. I agree with him completely. I suggest that any of you who haven't read the papers in question do so. Rodney has been asked to go over them with the entire Search Committee tomorrow. Ordinarily I would have thought that once that was done the committee would give Amstel short shrift. Now, I don't feel at all certain. For reasons I can't fathom, a candidate I felt the committee was indifferent to but a few days ago has the committee rallying around him out of all proportion to his worth."

"Surely you don't seriously think they intend to bring him here as head?" Bob Mettlar asked.

"I'm not at all confident they won't," Jim answered Bob just slowly shook his head.

"What can we do about it?" a junior member asked.

"In theory, we have nothing to say about it," answered Tony Lewis, "Jim here, gets his one vote on the committee of six, and can do his best to bring the others to his view of things."

"You mean we are completely helpless?" the same junior member asked.

"I said 'in theory'", Tony went on. "We can rally the opinion of others on the faculty. And if you have any influence with the politically powerful on the faculty, use it. Personally I am afraid I've used up most of my influence in past battles."

Bob Mettlar had been sitting grim faced during the last exchange. Now he rose and, facing Jim Kulp said quietly, but with intensity, "A former head should have little to say about his successor, and up to now I have not interfered." He paused choosing his next words. "The scientific literature ought to be sacred, It will be around long after its contributors are gone. To consider a man who appears, by his own publications, to hold it in such low esteem as the head for a scientific department is unthinkable. I shall go see Dean Mackenzie."

"Please don't, Bob, not yet at any rate," pleaded Jim "I'm not ready to admit to the rest of the Search Committee that we've had this meeting or our Sunday meeting with Dr. Mary White. I think that information would only infuriate the committee. Let's see how they respond to Rodney's session with them; then, if Rodney and I can't influence them, other approaches can be tried."

Professor Mettlar did not respond. He continued to look grim.

"Bob, I have to agree with Jim," Tony Lewis said. "Let's try honey first."

Mettlar did not look convinced. His complete silence was disconcerting and lay heavily on the entire proceedings.

As there was little else to discuss, the meeting slowly fragmented and Jim went to Tony's office where the conversation continued. Jim went into some detail concerning his visit with John Block and Dick Shane on the previous day.

"What did he mean by boy scout?" Tony asked, "I understand nit picker."

"I suppose he must have meant honor, a rigid regard for the truth," Jim speculated. "I don't know what else he could have been referring to."

Tony laughed "It seems two things a good investigator ought to be are a nit picker and a boy scout. You've been complimented."

"I agree, but I'm sure it wasn't meant that way. Tony, to change the subject, have you had any luck obtaining a commitment for funds from the Dean that I can use to support my work if my grant isn't renewed?"

"Not yet, Jim. I haven't given up but I'm not optimistic. Frank has been encouraging, perhaps even pressuring, department heads to obtain more and more money from outside grants. While I agree entirely with outside grants paying for research expenses, I don't like the trend toward paying faculty salaries from research funds. It is, unfortunately, a way in which the federal government can subsidize medical education with the least red tape. Medical research is like motherhood and available funds relatively easy to get."

"What happens when too many faculty members lose grants at the same time? Who'll pay their salaries?" Jim asked.

"That situation acts as a strong impetus not to lose a grant."

"You're telling me! I've worked hard at my research and have written it up, but getting it published is a problem. I'm afraid the people who pass on grants renewals and awards are like our Search Committee. They count publications. It's easier than reading them."

"Your problem is worse than that, Jim. You haven't given them one to count or read." Seeing the unhappy expression his words had produced on Jim's face, Tony rapidly went on, "You chose a difficult problem to solve. Certainly a worthwhile one; but nevertheless, a problem that wasn't apt to produce publications readily. Now you are suffering from that choice."

"It's ironic that to be successful one must be concerned more about the trappings of research than the research problem itself. Amstel is a beautiful example. I doubt he has any trouble getting grants," Jim said while shaking his head.

"What's more, he's editor-in-chief of a well known and read journal. Turning down his grant applications would be suicide if you wanted to publish in his journal." Tony's remark sparked the same thought in both their minds. They grinned at each other. "Well, have you considered sending your work to his journal?" Tony asked.

"My work could fit in it," he mused; but I don't need any more complications than this search has already produced. I must say I'm curious to see how Rodney fares with the Search Committee. He's much more at home with the subject of Amstel's research than I and should be more convincing. I don't see how they will be able to ignore the serious nature of the shortcomings those publications point out. It's not as though we were rejecting Amstel for personal reasons."

Tony thought for a moment and replied. "The problem may be that under ordinary circumstances, we, the department, would have no say in the matter. The Search Committee might well resent it if they perceived the department as trying to dictate the actions of the Committee."

Linda Koster stood in the preparation room to one side of the dialysis clinic. The patients on the morning shift were well into their six hour treatments and all was well. This was one Monday Linda desperately hoped it would be as she was in no mood for complications. Her life had suddenly taken an unsettling turn and its control was less hers than she was used to or wanted. The weekend affair, though far from common, was not unknown to her; but never before had it involved a spouse of one of her charges. Her professionalism had taken a beating in her own estimation, for if Linda was demanding of her co-workers, she was more so of herself. Even the faint suspicion that Marie Barret might approve of Linda performing her wifely duties for her did not lessen the self-dissatisfaction she was experiencing. She could not understand why she had allowed herself to behave as she did. Rodney was attractive, but she had been equally attracted to many other males and she was not particularly promiscuous. She partially blamed the alcohol they had imbibed, but she was well aware of the risks involved before her intake got out of hand.

She was lately aware of a growing desire to escape the reality of the demanding specialty she had chosen. She was fiercely proud of her ability to run her unit well. Her mastery of these complex techniques gave her a prestige she could not obtain elsewhere the hospital. The physicians needed the dialysis service, but few were as conversant with the numerous technical details as she. They were happy to rely on her expertise and would often defer to her judgments. Therein lay one attraction of her specialty.

Her patients, and with time they became hers, grew to depend on her and their evident worship bathed her ego like water the roots of a partially dried up plant. When they were doing well, she flourished; when they did poorly, she drooped. This metamorphosis took place under a seemingly thick outer skin and might be apparent to the astute observer only by the manner in which Linda treated he co-workers. On good days, she tended to be less sarcastic, less demanding and less desirous of making it thoroughly clear who was in charge of this unit. Despite this, or perhaps because of it, Linda was well respected in the hospital. Serious nurses enjoyed being on her service and often gained a degree of self-respect they had not previously felt. The house staff, often outwardly blasé, courted her good opinion and enjoyed seeing some of their less conscientious members suffer Linda's wrath. Their "Koster-rating" became an only semi-facetious in-joke among them. In view of the genuine rewards her position gave her, the signs she was detecting of a strong desire to escape, sorely troubled her. She could only explain the weekend in those terms. It was hard to be concerned about your patients when your physical senses are being acutely stimulated by other pursuits or your concerns deadened by alcohol. Her meditation was interrupted by the buzzing of an alarm on one of the consoles. She moved rapidly into the body of the unit and spotted the blinking light on the offending machine. It was a minor technical matter requiring an adjustment on a gauge, but it brought her to Marie Barret's vicinity.

"Did you enjoy the picnic?" Marie asked.

Linda appeared not to hear the question and Marie asked it again somewhat louder.

"I'm sorry, Marie, my mind was on that pressure gauge. It doesn't seem to be calibrated properly. Jeffrey," she called.

The dialysis technician came across the unit, and she conversed with him for a short time.

"The picnic, oh they're always fun. Such a perfect day. It seems the last few years we've had some rain."

"Did you see Rodney there?" Marie asked.

"Oh yes. He seemed very upset about something." Does Marie suspect? I wonder what Rodney told her to explain his absence, she thought.

"He's involved in departmental politics. They are choosing a new head for his department," Marie explained.

"I had heard. Guess they have been looking for several months now. Those searches are always painful for department members. It can really affect their futures."

"Rodney has tenure so he couldn't be fired without good reason, but there are other ways a new head can get rid of the incumbent faculty if he so chooses: take away space, give excessive teaching loads, make them generally miserable."

"Does that actually happen?"

"I've been told it does."

"Sounds like children, not grown men."

"They are children." Marie lay back in her chair and closed her eyes. "They need care," she said.

The latter statement and the way in which it was said struck Linda as though Marie might be turning Rodney over to her for safekeeping. She could not be cerftain it wasn't her own confusion reading meaning into Marie's words. She could not ask Marie directly, and she realized that if that was Marie's intent, she would continue to try and make her wishes known. Patients who felt their time had come often did concern themselves with their spouse's future. Linda continued her train of thought and wondered whether she would want Rodney were he to be bestowed upon her. To her, their weekend encounter had been enjoyable, even quite interesting, but she had not for a moment considered a serious alliance. What were her feelings toward Rodney? For that matter, what were her feelings toward a serious alliance with any man?

Dr. Barret was waiting outside the small clinical classroom that Dr. Block had been able to reserve on such short notice for their meeting. The entire Search Committee was inside. A classroom had been chosen to give Rodney Barret a chalkboard for his presentation. This sudden meeting had to be scheduled for the early morning to interfere least with the previous plans of the men involved. John Block briefly sketched the weekend's activities for the entire committee and concluded, "In view of the seriousness of the allegations concerning Dr. Amstels scientific abilities, we felt you should have the opportunity to hear for yourselves from Dr. Barret the nature of the complaints. We've asked him to give us his views and he is outside waiting to do so. Before we have him in, are there comments anyone cares to make?"

Professor Lawrence Root scowled. "I do not understand this, John. What has Dr. Barret to do with the deliberations of this Search Committee?"

"I asked Rodney to speak to us Larry, because his field of expertise is most closely related to that of the candidate. The fact that Rodney is in the Pharmacology department is coincidental."

"I still don't like it. This committee is in no way responsible to Pharmacology."

Jim Kulp broke in. "We are responsible to the school and should make the best choice possible."

"I do not need you to remind me of that, young man," answered Professor Root giving Jim a withering scowl.

"Gentlemen, let us keep our discussions on a scientific plane. Shall we hear the evidence?" John asked.

No one answered so he went to the door and brought Rodney into the room. As he was doing this a scraping sound was heard as Professor Root was turning his chair around so that his back faced the chalkboard and Dr. Barret. He remained in that position throughout Rodney's presentation which was informal and sprinkled with a few questions from the committee. When he came to the part concerning the control data for the male and female mouse experiment, John Block pursued the same line of questioning he had with Jim Kulp. Jim was overjoyed, because on reflection he felt no one would believe his story that John Block, the eminent investigator, could be that naive about biological data. Now here he was in front of all these people pursuing the same course.

"Dr. Barret, is there no chance those control data were obtained from two experiments, one on male and one on female mice?" John asked.

"There is a chance," Rodney answered and John began to beam. "But it's less than one chance in six trillion experiments." John's smile faded and was replaced by a grim stare.

Professor Evans asked Rodney about the solvents Amstel had used in his extractions and agreed that some of the choices were inappropriate. His questions led Jim to suspect he was much less qualified to discuss this research field than was Rodney Barret although, of the committee members, his research was the closest to Amstel's and he was considered by the committee an expert in that field.

When the presentation was over Rodney was coolly thanked and dismissed. As he left the scraping sound occurred again and Professor Root once again faced forward. His face was flushed.

"In all my experience, I have never known such a shocking breach of protocol," he said. "To have a member of the department for which we are selecting a head excoriate one of our candidates," he stopped, clearly unable to choose the next words to express his anger.

"That is unfair," retorted Jim, "Rodney came here because we asked him. He was concerned when he heard Amstel was coming for a second visit."

"Are you saying, Dr. Kulp, that someone on this committee, you, for instance, has ignored our charge to meet in executive session? You have actually divulged the deliberations of this group?" Professor Root had now turned his wrathful countenance on Jim.

Jim's first inclination was to deny informing Rodney of Amstels second visit as he had not done so. Instead, he almost shouted, "I don't intend to keep information from my department which can serve to allay their fears during this period of intense disruption."

"This is shocking!" exclaimed Professor Root in a markedly pompous manner. The room was silent.

Jim, who had regained his composure stated, "I differ from some members of this committee."

"And, how pray tell?" asked Professor Root.

Jim looked at each member of the committee and quietly said, "At least, I tell the truth." His remark was ignored by all and served only to relieve some of his frustration.

Harry Tatum, who up to this point in the meeting had been silent now spoke. "These criticisms of Dr. Amstel's papers—I find this disturbing. Especially this business about the male and female controls. A question of integrity is raised in my mind which really disturbs me. Could we get a second opinion on these publications from someone not in Pharmacology or on the committee?"

"That sounds reasonable. Whom do you suggest?" asked John.

"What about Mary White? Surely none of us would question her integrity or ability," Harry said. A feeling of intense relief bordering on joy filled Jim Kulp.

"I don't like the idea of every Tom, Dick and Harry meddling in our affairs." Professor Root objected.

"I can't agree with you Larry," John came to the rescue. "If a majority of the committee concur, I think Harry's suggestion is a good one." He looked around and only Professor Root protested. "Ill set up a meeting with Mary as soon as possible." He rose and quickly left the room.

Later in the week, Professor Mary White met with the committee. The results were similar except that Professor Root did not turn his back this time, but neither did he open his mouth. Dr. White deplored the sorry state of the publications from a strictly scientific point of view. After she left the meeting, Jim Kulp sensed a disturbing change in the deliberations. Now instead of trying to deny the inadequacy of the candidates scientific abilities, his other virtues were being stressed. Dick Shane pointed out that the Wilder staff included no editors of prestigious journals. The candidates political abilities and their value in helping to build up the department were stressed.

"I wouldn't care if Sidney Amstel had never written a paper," Jim stated, "I'd be all for him if he hadn't published those."

The remarks of Harry Tatum of Pathology, set the stage for subsequent events. "The critiques of Amstel's papers have raised serious questions. These questions must be resolved before I could vote on whether or not to offer the Chairmanship to Dr. Amstel."

"The only way to do that would be to question the candidate himself," John Block allowed. "Who would do that?"

"Not our department," Jim volunteered, "they've already informed me of that."

"That leaves it up to the committee," said John. "Dr. Amstel is slated to visit in two weeks. We can do it then."

Jim suddenly realized that Amstel had already been invited for a second visit. He wondered when he had been invited. Perhaps the very moment after the committee had voted for him that Saturday morning before the student faculty picnic. That would help explain the extreme resistance he encountered on his visit with Block and Shane that Sunday. They were embarrassed and reacting to their own blunder. That must be it, he guessed, but where do we go from here?

Andy Beardsley's third-year clinical clerkship on Obstetrics had finished months previously, and he was presently doing his stint on Pediatrics. He enjoyed working with the children, but was saddened by the crippling diseases and those with a fatal outcome more so than he had been on adult services. As yet he had not decided which, if any, specialty he preferred; that decision would come later in the fourth year.

By his classmates, Andy was perceived to be calm, unflappable, easygoing. Academically, he was slightly above average. He now seemed preoccupied and spent more of his all too precious free time brooding. None of Donna's probing produced satisfactory answers, but she was certain something was wrong The initial signs she felt had begun while he was on Obstetrics. She knew he enjoyed the work on that clerkship and received a respectable grade, which made the situation puzzling.

Their home life, what little there was of it, was essentially a happy one. They shared a rich enjoyment of their offspring and, as is often the case with busy people, had little time for the minor annoyances which can play havoc with relationships where people do not have enough to do. Andy, who previously had always slept well, was having trouble sleeping. He would either have difficulty going to sleep or would awaken in the middle of the night.

The evening of the day Dr. Kulp's laboratory finished and sent off the publication, they hoped for the last time, she felt like celebrating. She had bought a bottle of red wine, cooked an especially tasty supper and dined with Andy by candle light. After supper they danced to radio music, made love and drifted off to sleep especially relaxed. Soon after midnight Donna was awakened by Andy who made strange noises as though he were crying. When awake enough to comprehend what was happening, she realized Andy was having a nightmare. He became agitated and began moaning in his sleep. "Don't, don't, please don't!" and then he would weep. Donna became alarmed and shook him until he awoke. He looked so dejected she hated herself for being cross with him, but she demanded, "Andy, what is wrong with you? What were you dreaming about?"

He sat on the edge of the bed not saying a word but staring at the wall. Donna turned on a light and sat watching him. Finally he turned to her with tears streaming down his face and kissed her.

"I have got to tell someone for my sanity, but I hate to burden you with my dilemma, still I don't know who else I can tell. Worse still, I don't know how to resolve the problem."

"Why don't you tell me about it?" Donna coaxed as she held him.

"Now that I am about to tell you, I suddenly feel as though I've been making a mountain out of a mole hill. I feel silly?"

"Tell me Andy. What's the problem? You don't usually get emotional for no reason."

"Your right. Okay," He sighed. "When I was on obstetrics you remember the students took turns taking all-night duty to learn to deliver babies. Well, one night when I was on, we delivered a baby about three in the morning for an indigent mother. All was going smoothly. The baby's head appeared, the shoulders followed and what seemed a normal delivery seemed to suddenly stop. Dr. Krecke, a resident, was there. He took over for me and soon found the trouble. The baby had a meningocele at the base of its spine and this was slowing the delivery. He and I were the only observers present. The nurse was out of the delivery room. When the delivery was finished, Krecke carried the baby to the next room. I stayed with the mother applying external pressure to her abdomen to limit bleeding from the uterus. That seems to be a chore reserved for medical students. The mother was exhausted and fell asleep never having seen her baby with the large mass on its spine. I thought Krecke had taken it off to examine it out of the mother's presence before he broke the news to her. After a few minutes, the nurse came back so I got her to hold the uterus as I was curious to see the meningocele more closely. I went into the next room in time to see Krecke trying to drown the baby in the sink. When he saw me he said the baby would require extensive surgery and years to repair and might never be right. There was no way these parents could afford that. He was doing them a favor. They'd have others. He told me to get out! I did, but as I left I could hear the baby. There was nothing wrong with its lungs. I can still hear it. Tonight I was back in that room with Krecke and the baby. That dream was so real."

"Oh Andy, how horrible. Well, what or how was it reported on the chart? What story was given the mother?"

"They called it stillborn. No one even questioned it."

"Have you discussed it with Krecke?"

"No, not a word. It's as though it never happened. When I speak of it now, it might all have been a dream. I looked up meningocele in the library. Some are very extensive and do cause serious neurological problems; others are minor. I don't know how good a diagnostician Krecke is. He could have been entirely wrong in his estimate of the situation."

"He can't kill a baby no matter what!"

"He did."

"What are you going to do?"

"After all this time, I don't know. I couldn't bring myself to report it then. I've vacillated between condoning his actions as proper and thinking him a madman who shouldn't be loose on the public. He has a good reputation and may well be the next chief resident on Obstetrics."

"You ought to report him."

"I'd ruin his career, probably my own, since the unwritten law says you don't rat on fellow physicians. I'd made up my mind to forget it, but I obviously can't. Telling now would not bring the baby back. I don't know whether the meningocele was dissected out in pathology. I've almost gone to look it up, but if Krecke was wrong I don't want to know it."

"No wonder you've been disturbed lately."

"Honey," he kissed her, "telling you has made me feel better already. Let's assume it was a bad dream and try and forget it."

They turned off the light and soon Donna could tell that Andy had fallen off to sleep. She lay awake thinking of the horrid tale she had just heard. Relieved to know the origin of Andy's odd behavior, she was saddened to think that such things went on and that Andy, no matter how remotely, was part of them. She wondered how long it would take her to calm down and whether she would sleep well at night.

"But we can't break it to him that way, John." Jim Kulp was in John Block's office. "Amstel is bringing his wife along to look for housing. As far as Amstel is concerned, he feels the ball is mostly in his court now. He'll listen to the Dean's offer, negotiate and decide. You know a second visit usually means he's got the job if he wants it."

"That's true."

"Well, how would you feel if you took your wife to look at a supposedly sure thing and they sat you down to an embarrassing confrontation?"

"You have a point, Jim, What do you propose?"

Encouraged, as this was the first time since the search had started that Jim felt he really had John's attention, he continued. "If we were to call Amstel at his home this evening and tell him the truth, he'd have several days in which to make a decision before he's scheduled to fly down here. In the seclusion of his own home, he can think it over, call us and tell us to 'get lost' he's decided against considering Wilder. He can then tell his associates he has decided against this job. He doesn't lose face. He needn't even tell his wife his real reasons. As far as anyone knows, it was his decision, not ours, to call it off. That makes more sense. Breaking it to him when he arrives is cruel!"

John listened and was quiet for several moments after Jim finished his plea. "There's some merit to what you propose."

Some merit, thought Jim, any other course at this point is ridiculous. He was beginning to learn the wisdom of holding his tongue.

"Since we have little time left," John continued, "I'll call a meeting of the committee at my home this evening and we can discuss it then."

Jim was disappointed that John did not simply call Amstel himself that evening without involving the entire Search Committee. His plan he thought was so simple and under the circumstances, intelligent, that considerate human beings would have no other choice.

The faculty of the Pharmacology Department were in their small library. Jim had assembled the group to pass on information regarding the latest developments.

"I can't understand the thinking of these people," he told them. "We met for three hours last night just to consider whether we should call Amstel at his home and warn him what was in store for him on this visit. You would have been proud of me. I was quiet, polite and I am sure they could not read my thoughts."

"That must have been a great strain on you," said Rodney laughing.

"But those dimwits, they actually decided that calling him and telling him on the phone was too 'impersonal'. They'll tell him when he arrives. Can you believe that?"

Incredulity was widely expressed.

"I'm tempted to call him myself. I think what they are doing is cruel. You just don't treat people that way!"

"Your motives would be misunderstood," Bob Mettlar asserted.

"I agree. That's the thing that keeps me from phoning Amstel," Jim answered.

"How do they plan to confront him?" Tony Lewis asked.

"I don't know. That hasn't been discussed in my presence. They may have been meeting without me. I don't think they appreciated me saying I'd not respect secrecy if in so doing I could avoid undue strain on all of you."

We appreciate that, Jim," Bob Mettlar said thoughtfully, "but you do have a duty to the committee and I do not believe you should neglect it."

"Hell, I don't care if they kick me off the committee."

"Then we'd have no support," Rodney Barret countered. "That would be dumb. Stay with the committee, restrain your natural impulses. It will build character," he chortled.

"What is expected of us on this visit?" asked Tony Lewis.

"I suppose Amstel will want to talk with each of us. After all, as far as he knows, he'll be our new chief."

"This is a childish charade," said Bob Mettlar.

"What else can we do? We don't want to appear hostile or rude. He's pleasant enough to talk to and, aside from his behavior as a scientist, I have nothing against him," Jim asserted.

"Do you suppose they'll seriously try to bring him here as head?" asked Tony.

"They must mean to offer him the chairmanship," answered Jim. "I gave them what I thought was an easy way out of a difficult situation. No one would have been embarrassed. We could have continued searching. Since they didn't take it I assume they think it is a done deal. Harry Tatum is the only one who expressed a need to have the published discrepancies explained away before he could vote to bring him here. That suggests the others don't care. At best that means a four to two vote by the committee for him will go to the Dean."

"He still has to get past the Executive Committee," added Tony.

"Is that binding or merely advisory to the Dean?" asked Rodney.

"Strictly speaking, it is purely advisory," answered Bob Mettlar, "but in such matters the Dean usually listens to his department heads."

"Bob, do you think we could get enough of the department chairman on our side to swing the Executive Committee to our way of thinking?" Jim asked.

"I don't know," Bob Mettlar answered, "but if the Dean wants this man badly enough, he as Dean has ways to influence the Executive Committee with which we would find it difficult to compete. I am not certain how the Dean stands in all this."

"Professor Root felt he had impressed the Dean and so did Dick Shane. The Dean must be for him, though I don't know how strongly," Jim asserted. After a period of silence he continued. "That is all the information I have for you. I'll keep you informed though I doubt anything will happen between now and Amstel's visit." The group disbursed.

Jim went back to his laboratory to find Bill Michaelson counting samples of radioactive-labeled insulin with a Geiger counter and scaler.

"How's the work going?" he asked.

"Fine, Dr. Kulp. I'm just finishing up that separation experiment we did earlier this week"

"Aren't you going to be late for obstetrical rounds, Bill? Jake Bourne won't care for that."

Bill glanced at his watch. "I guess so, but I want to finish these soon. I've got others coming off the column now and I don't want to get too far behind."

"I'm free all afternoon. Let me count them for you." Jim thought some lab work would be good occupational therapy as a diversion from his committee work. Bill appreciated the offer and acquiesced. Jim sat by the equipment and counted one sample after the other and recorded the results. As he was familiar with the experiment he was not at all happy with the results he was getting from the counter. When the samples which should have been high in radioactivity had their procedure gone well, the scaler was blinking at a frustrating slow rate. Isn't anything going right? he thought. In disgust, he pulled the holder and sample out of its counting position and away from the Geiger tube. Ordinarily the scaler would have stopped blinking. It didn't. If anything, it blinked faster. Jim sat staring at the scaler. What's going on? he wondered.

The Geiger tube and scaler were on a laboratory bench against the front wall of the medical school building. From where he sat he could look out the front windows. He picked up a piece of lead shielding used to block radiation and placed it over the counting end of the Geiger tube. The scaler stopped counting. My God, he thought, is this whole bench contaminated with radioactivity? He picked up the Geiger tube which resembled a flashlight with a wire attaching it to the scaler. He pointed it at various portions of the laboratory desk and quickly noted the counting grew higher as he approached the window. These counts, too, were stopped by the lead shield. As he looked out of the window, he remembered that a gentle rain had been falling but moments before. He had heard news reports from time to time of atomic testing out West, but that was miles away and he had heard nothing recently.

"God damn Eisenhower," he said aloud. He thought frantically, what shall I do? This can't be. Maybe the equipment is at fault. He knew he could quickly check the scaler. There was a similar one upstairs in Biochemistry he had used from time to time. He detached the Geiger tube and ran upstairs. There the same phenomena occurred though the counts were lower. Of course, he thought, we're further from the ground and that's where the radioactivity is coming from. It must have come down with the rain. He returned to his office, picked up the phone and called home.

"Honey," he asked when Janet picked up the phone, "Where are the children?"

"Out playing in the yard. Why?"

"Bring them inside and keep them there until you hear from me!"

"Why, Jim?"

"I'll tell you later, just do it please. Oh, and remove their clothing and give them baths."

"What's going on?" she was alarmed.

"Don't say anything to anybody yet, but I think we've had some fall out from a radioactive cloud with the rain. It has rained there, hasn't it?

"Not yet. Looks threatening though."

"That's good. Get them in before it does. Call you later." He hung up and called the radiation laboratory in the Public Health School across the street. He spoke with an acquaintance there, related his experience, and his friend agreed to check immediately. He returned to the original scaler, reattached the Geiger tube and checked again. The counts continued, though at a slower rate, he thought. He hadn't done a full count or recorded any of the results.

Should I call the State Police? What should I say to them? This could cause a panic. Is all this a bad dream? By now he could see through the window that his friend with the battery-operated portable counting unit was scanning the ground. He soon appeared in the laboratory and tended to confirm Jim's findings. Yes, the counts were above the normal background for cosmic radiation. The two were discussing what to do next when Rodney Barret entered the room. He noted the worried looks and asked about them. Jim told him. Rodney went through the maneuvers Jim described with similar results. Rodney, however, went further. He pointed the Geiger tube towards a fluorescent ceiling lamp and the scaler went crazy with counts. He then inserted a piece of cardboard as Jim had inserted the lead. The counting stopped.

He laughed, "You've been counting radiation all right. It's just not atomic in origin. How long have you had that Geiger tube?"

"Several years," Jim answered.

"With age, some Geiger tubes become light sensitive." Rodney explained. That's the problem.

Jim was at once intensely relieved and chagrined.

"Thank God I didn't call the police or spread this around." As he considered what might have happened he cringed. What a time to make a complete ass of myself, he thought. I'd better call Janet.

That humbling experience made Jim even more concerned about the events which were to befall Sidney Amstel. He was more able to put himself in Sidney's shoes. He would, for example, far prefer to avoid the issue completely than to have to explain to a panel of his peers why he called the State Police and caused havoc had he done so. It was lucky Rodney came in when he did.

What he couldn't explain was his friend from across the street's corroboration. It must have been the power of suggestion, he thought before dismissing the whole episode from his mind.

Marie Barret's thinking was in turmoil. Her intense faith and rigid adherence to Catholic doctrine made any serious thought of suicide unacceptable. The thought that she would slowly fade away and die and her calm acceptance of that without an intentional struggle, had begun to give her guilt feelings. Was this not similar to suicide?

As her condition seemed to stabilize. she slowly began to adjust to the thrice weekly dialysis sessions. She became an accepted member of the group of patients and was slowly taking an interest in their individual problems. She even thought of planning ways to make their common condition the source of something positive: perhaps a local chapter of dialysis recipients helping each other within some organizational structure. Marie was an organizer and to be truly happy had to feel productive. The demands of her children did, in truth, require all her restricted energies, yet for some reason were not fulfilling. Her beginning estrangement from Rodney was very upsetting and at the same time a relief in that it assuaged her guilt over her flagging sexual desire. Any thought that Rodney might be unfaithful she drove from her mind—not because of the effect on her ego, but because she considered such, unworthy for those of her faith. Rodney was too perfect to sin. Yet deep down, she knew something had occurred when Rodney stayed away all night. She did suspect that Linda might have been his partner and was strangely not jealous. She was, however disappointed to think Linda would take advantage of the nurse/patient relationship. Another part of her sought a substitute to aid Rodney and her family were she to die. She respected and liked Linda, and her suspicions were just suspicions. She was incensed to learn that the committee seemed to be rejecting Rodney as a choice for department head. She knew that a new head would eventually mean Rodney would seek employment elsewhere. Previously, a move would have been exciting for her, particularly if it enhanced his career. Now a move meant a new dialysis unit. First, she would have to be accepted on the favored list. Her problems rather than Rodney's might dictate where they would go and this she found hard to accept. She always subordinated her desires to Rodney's career of which she was extremely protective and proud. What could she do? How could she cope?

She was in this confused and depressed state of mind when Rodney informed her of Amstel's second visit and the fact that their presence was requested at a dinner party for the visitor and his wife to be held at Dean Mackenzie's later in the week. Though she could beg off and would have on the grounds of her condition, she was curious to see the man who was being chosen in Rodney's stead. In addition, she had very little social life of late, and previous parties at the Dean's had been fun owing to the Herculean efforts of his wife Millicent. Most of the Pharmacology

Department would be present and she enjoyed the faculty wives. Much to Rodney's surprise she accepted the invitation and was now seriously concerned over what she would wear. The evening undoubtedly would be warm, but her shunt dictated a long sleeve dress or the visibility of an unsightly bandage. Rodney marveled at the human psyche. One minute life-and-death decisions, and then, with no less intensity, sartorial problems.

The morning of Dr. Amstel's arrival on campus, Rodney had decided to sleep late. For him to do so on a weekday morning was unusual. He was escaping. Not knowing what to expect he wanted to sleep through all he could. Shortly after ten, he heard the phone ring and could hear Marie answering. The silence which followed convinced him of impending trouble and he snuggled deeper in the bedclothes though the room was warm from the morning sun. Marie, who was usually solicitous brusquely entered.

"Pick up the phone,Rod, it's Jim." He groaned but did as he was told.

Rodney, where the hell are you?" Jim's voice was frantic.

"In bed, where else?" Rodney chortled.

"Can you get down here right away? We've got to quiz Dr. Amstel."

"I thought your committee was going to do that."

"We were, but Amstel insisted he be confronted by his accusers. He's taking it amazingly well." Rodney was silent. Jim went on. "You still there?"

"Yeah."

"Shane brought him to my office about half an hour ago, and he told me he didn't want to deal second hand. I asked who he would like going over his papers; and he suggested you, Bob and me. I told him I'd hate to be quizzed on a publication I authored on such short notice and to take some time to refresh his memory, but he declined. We'll meet in Bob's office as soon as you can get here. Bring along your copies. How long will you be?"

"Three-quarters of an hour, but I'd like to not come at all."

"You're not alone in that. I figured I'd be in on it no matter who did it, but I didn't expect this."

"Do you suppose Shane put him up to it?"

"Don't know."

"See you soon." Rodney hung up and slowly rose from the bed. He showered, dressed and had his morning coffee all the time dreading the chore he was to undertake. He thought about accusers and whistle blowers who often appear more villainous than the villains. Where Science was concerned, Rodney allowed no imperfections, yet he enjoyed popularity and was unhappy in a censorious role.

He arrived at work in time to catch Professor Mettlar, Dr. Amstel and Jim Kulp coming back from coffee in the hospital cafeteria. They closeted themselves in Bob's office around a small conference table with firm instructions not to be disturbed. Copies of the publications in question were spread on the table. After a minimum of "small talk," they proceeded to the business at hand. The three Wilderians were amazed at Amstel's poise. He seemed, if anything, trying to make their job easy, almost enjoyable. They would point out errors and Amstel would acknowledge them.

"The solvent used in this extraction—wouldn't it react with the material you wanted to extract and measure, and thus make the measurement faulty?" Bob Mettlar asked.

"I realized that as soon as I'd done the experiment," Amstel admitted.

"Then why did you publish it?" asked Rodney.

"I didn't want to," said Amstel, "but my co-authors talked me into it."

After a few moments of complete silence Rodney continued. "The two tables in this paper," he said holding up the copy, "they're mathematical transpositions of the same data. I guess you wanted to look at the data in two different ways. At any rate, we did the conversions on a calculator. Of twenty conversions, fifteen in your published paper are wrong. Granted some of these are small errors, but some are off by over fifty percent and others by an order of magnitude."

Amstel studied the tables for a few seconds and a sheet of paper Rodney handed him with the calculations on it. He appeared relaxed compared to the grim demeanor of the others. He finally looked up and smiled. "I guess I should have used a calculator."

When they pointed out the discrepancy concerning the control data for the male and female mouse papers Amstel readily admitted the published controls were from the same animals, but he was genuinely perplexed and kept saying, "I don't understand. I know we had the appropriate control data."

The rapidity with which Amstel understood and accepted their criticisms made them suspect that he had been through this exercise before. They did not think the committee was responsible since there had not been time, but someone must have pointed out these errors to him some time in the past. He was so well conversant with them.

When they had finished going over the papers, Dr. Amstel asked if he might visit alone with Dr. Mettlar. Rodney and Jim excused themselves overjoyed to depart.

"I want to ask you some questions about departmental budgets and the like," Amstel said. He rose and reached across the table sweeping up the copies of his papers which lay there. He stacked them neatly and placed them in his briefcase, closed it and said matter-of-factly. "Oh well, chickens will come home to roost!"

Jim Kulp went to his office to await the finish of Amstel's talk with Professor Mettlar. He was then to deliver Sidney to Dick Shane who was to take him to lunch. As he waited, he tried to do some work but his mind would not concentrate on any subject other than Amstel. He marveled at the man's composure and was nearly euphoric at the apparent ease with which an embarrassing undertaking had been accomplished. Soon Amstel came in and sat.

"Did you have a good chat with Bob?"

"Yes. He answered my questions, Jim," and looking directly at him asked, "How did you feel I did?"

Jim shook his head. "Sid, emotionally, I am all for you, but intellectually I can't excuse your behavior as a scientist." Then, tired of feeling guilty for Amstel's transgressions, he asked, "What do you think B.J. would think of all this?" B.J. was the former chief of the Pharmacology Department where Sidney Amstel and James Kulp had both received their graduate degrees. He was a good scientist and had the reputation for extremely careful work.

"I know exactly what B.J. would have thought," Amstel replied, "but you know Jim, there are very few fastidious scientists in this country, and they don't count for much."

At that moment, Jim, who had been feeling quite sympathetic toward and obliged to Sidney for making the interview so painless, lost all respect for the man. If anything, Amstel's last remark erased in Jim most of the guilt concerning the gauche way in which this whole affair had been handled by the committee.

Bill Michaelson was not enjoying his first few days on Obstetrics. Through no fault of his own he had gotten off to a bad start. Some secretary in the Dean's office had made an error in the scheduling sent him and he missed the introductory lecture given his group in which the workings of their time on Obstetrics were explained and assignment schedules for night duty were made. When he finally reported to the resident in charge, the situation worsened. Dr. Krecke refused to recognize that Bill had been other than dilatory in missing the first lecture. He resented having to spend the time giving Bill course details and his night schedule, and he was practically apoplectic at Bill's suggestion of a minor modification which would have made Bill's clinical and work schedules mesh conveniently. Ever since, he had taken every possible opportunity to berate Bill in public for minor errors: the kind invariably made by students with new and unfamiliar techniques. It was obvious to Bill that he was to be the goat of his group of students. Unfortunately, this minor harassment, which most intelligent students would have ignored and tolerated produced in Bill a mixed reaction. It made him nervous and further hindered his performance. In addition, he resented his unfair treatment and made the mistake of responding to Krecke's barbs with barbs of his own. Krecke's ego would not tolerate this from a subordinate and he fully intended to put this upstart student in his place.

In obstetrics, as in all of medicine, there are routine, time-consuming jobs which must be done, But once mastered are just plain dull. Such jobs usually fall to the medical students to perform. In addition, there are chores which by their nature tend to be unpleasant. These, too, are delegated to the lowest members of the medical hierarchy. Krecke made sure that, if at all possible, every such job or chore was assigned to Bill. When interesting things were happening on the service, Krecke tried to see that Bill was busily employed with some of this "scut work". Bill was thoroughly frustrated.

One evening before the medical students left the wards, a complicated delivery was in progress. The baby was not progressing normally through the birth canal resulting in a prolonged and exhausting delivery for the young mother. Krecke had examined the mother by reaching into the birth canal and feeling with his fingers. He pulled off his sterile gloves and had two medical students scrub, glove and gown and do similar inspections. Just as the last student was finishing, Bill returned from a routine chore. Krecke smiled and instructed Bill to examine the patient as well. Before Bill had returned, he had explained to the other students that the object they were feeling at the mouth of the uterus were the baby's toes and that he would have to deliver the baby feet first, a relatively difficult technical delivery but one with which he could cope. He was pleased to be able to show off his skills. Bill was unaware of any of this, and when he had finished his examination, Krecke was to have the added pleasure of quizzing him.

"Well, Doctor what do you make of that?" Krecke asked in his most sarcastic voice. Bill was silent and deep in thought. Krecke went on with relish. "What did you feel? You did feel something, didn't you?"

"I don't know."

"You don't know whether you felt something, Doctor?" The last word was accentuated.

"I felt something in the birth canal, but I'm not certain what it was," said Bill.

"Was it a head?" Krecke smiled at the other students.

"Obviously not," countered Bill whose annoyance was all to obvious.

Sensing he was losing his position of advantage in the eyes of the others present who now included some nurses and other house staff, Krecke became very businesslike and ignoring Bill, went on, "in footling cases like this it is important to…" but Bill interrupted firmly.

"In what cases?"

"Footling, the baby presenting with his feet coming out first," an annoyed Krecke answered.

"That was not a foot I felt," Bill stated flatly.

Krecke was unbelieving at this student's nerve. "What was it then?" he asked.

I don't know," Bill frowned.

"Well if you don't know, Doctor, I do so please stop interrupting. I would like those capable of learning here to get the chance free of your inane suggestions."

As Dr. Krecke was attempting to put Bill in his place, the patient had an especially strong contraction.

A nurse standing near the patient gasped, "Dr. Krecke Look!"

Protruding from the birth canal between its Mother's parted thighs was an outstretched hand.

"Damn," shouted Bill excitedly, "I knew it wasn't a foot, but why didn't I think of a hand!"

At this point, Dr. Krecke and the nurses flew into action.

Krecke lectured to the students as he rolled the bed towards the operating room.

"When an arm comes out of the birth canal pressure from the contracting uterus can cause all sorts of harm to the baby and necessitates rapid surgical intervention."

Within a very short time the patient was transferred to an operating table, prepped, draped and anesthetized. Quickly Dr. Krecke's skilled hands cut through the skin, fat and muscle of the abdomen and then through the muscle of the uterus from which he extracted a small red doll-like figure which was starting its first day outside of its mother.

When the excitement was over and the frantic activity stopped, Dr. Krecke was grim. In view of the success of the Cesarean delivery, his demeanor was puzzling and his short gruff answers to student's questions made it apparent that something was upsetting him. He did not recognize Bill's presence. He did not look at nor speak to him, and when Bill asked him a question, it appeared as if the question was unheard.

When the students had left the ward, they congratulated Bill on his diagnostic coup. Bill who felt stupid for not recognizing the hand he felt, was relieved not to have angered Krecke further by diagnosing the baby's true position earlier. One of the students was laughingly pointing out Bill's superiority to Krecke to a group of students he'd come upon in the cafeteria when Krecke entered and heard him. He pretended not to hear, but from the manner in which the color drained from his already grim face, it was obvious to those who saw him that something had happened. That damn student will never graduate if I can help it, he vowed to himself.

The evening was pleasantly warm. The smell of gardenias in the bushes which lined the walk to the Dean' house was delightful. The smooth conversion from Winter to Spring made this a particularly good year for gardenias. Janet remarked to Jim how hard she still found it to get used to all these gardenias on bushes. As a young girl living in the North, these had been her favorite corsage flower, and to see them in such abundance was unreal. Ahead on the path, Janet saw Marie and Rodney Barret who stopped and awaited their approach. Marie was wearing a sleeveless gown and had partially solved the shunt problem by hiding the bandage with long evening gloves and a large and pretty silk shawl around her shoulders and arms.

"You look lovely," remarked Janet.

"Thank you Jan, but I feel conspicuous," answered Marie.

"You needn't," said Jim and added quietly to Rodney, "Feeling better about things now the ordeal is over?"

"I don't think it's over. Far from it," Rodney replied.

"Stop talking shop, you two." demanded Janet. "Let's make this a pleasant evening."

"I'll second that," said Rodney as they walked into the Dean's house which was filled with guests milling about drinks in hand.

"So glad to see you," Millicent Mackenzie greeted them soon after they entered. "Dr. and Mrs. Amstel... Oh, excuse me, Dr. and Dr. Amstel, the guests of honor are in the far room," she motioned in the direction "They're receiving. We wanted everyone to get a chance to meet them tonight. The beverages are served in the opposite direction."

"Let's get a drink first," Rodney suggested, "it appears there are an abundance of "greeters" right now."

"You're just chicken," whispered Jim. "Both areas are crowded, but I'll bet there are many more at the refreshments."

"Let's get a drink," Rodney repeated.

"Nothing for me, thanks," said Marie who was restricting her fluid intake and had to pace herself carefully. The four of them drifted slowly across the house into the room where the guests of honor were holding forth. Mrs. Amstel was describing her tour that day in the hands of a local real estate agent who was a town character. The agent was extremely aggressive and this aggression combined with a degree of absentmindedness led to situations more amusing in the telling than the happening. In any case, it was plain to all who listened that Barbara Amstel was seriously house hunting. The Kulps and the Barrets greeted the Amstels, and to the casual observer none of the conflicts appeared on the surface to mar the enjoyment of the evening. Soon Dean Mackenzie joined the group and, playing the role of genial host, smiled more than Jim had witnessed in all his years at Wilder. It was apparent that Frank Mackenzie was wooing Sidney Amstel for the position and either did not know, or worse, did not care about his scientific transgressions. That realization tended to depress Jim and Rodney, and meeting the other members of their department did not help to elevate their moods.

The evening passed smoothly and no references veiled or otherwise passed to or from the candidate or the Pharmacology Department. If anything Amstel seemed to be taking a slightly parental attitude toward the department members as if his selection was a foregone conclusion.

At one point during the evening, Jim and Bob Mettlar were able to converse in private. "He seems almost certain he's a shoe-in, doesn't he?" Jim remarked.

"Yes, he does, Bob said slowly. His expression became stern. "Jim, I want you to tell Block something for me." His tone left little doubt in Jim's mind that he'd better listen carefully. "If he tries to bring that man here as department head, I'll go to the Dean. If I can't stop it there, I'll go to the Chancellor. If I can't get it stopped there, I'll go to the President, the Board of Trustees or the Governor and Legislature." Jim knew Bob was not bluffing.

Not long after John Block joined them and Bob Mettlar rapidly and not very subtly excused himself. Jim chose not to deliver his massage, feeling this was neither the time nor the place. John Block delivered news of his own. Monday afternoon the Search Committee was going to quiz Amstel on his papers. Professor Harry Tatum's concerns regarding the questions raised about Amstel were probably behind this second confrontation. Jim's mood continued to deteriorate as he realized he would have to sit through it all over again.

The following Monday morning an incident occurred, having nothing to do with choosing a department head, but which helped Jim Kulp and Rodney Barret keep their problems in perspective and their sanity intact. The departmental diener, who maintained all the equipment and paraphernalia used by the members in teaching and research was a twin named John Dewey Carlson. His brother James Louis Carlson was diener for the Physiology department. Early that morning John had phoned in to report he would be unable to come in today. He had to attend his grandfather's funeral. Jim Kulp, at the laboratory early to keep his research going smoothly, had taken John Dewey's call. At the time he was skeptical since the morning was a beautiful and John Dewey was an avid fisherman not above playing hooky. At coffee break time, James Louis, as was his wont, came from Physiology to James's shop to visit his twin brother. Unable to find him, he stuck his head through the open door of Jim Kulp's office where Jim and Rodney stood conversing, and asked if they'd seen his brother. A peculiar expression came over Jim's face.

"He's gone to his grandfather's funeral," he said. After a pause Jim bluntly asked, "You do have the same grandfather, don't you?"

James Louis looked confused and answered, "No."

For a moment there was complete silence. Then Jim Kulp began to laugh. Rodney, who didn't know of John Dewey's phone call, looked embarrassed and could not understand Jim Kulp's apparent callousness. Jim was laughing so hard he had difficulty standing and fell into the nearest chair holding his abdomen. John Dewey realized that his twin was playing hooky, and countered with the statement that James Louis must have meant his wife's grandfather had died; but, through choking laughter, Jim informed John Dewey that unless he had a new wife, he had already used that excuse twice before. Rodney now realized what was going on and joined in the mirth, though not so forcefully as Jim. James Louis, with a hurt look and his dignity not quite intact, took his leave from "The two mad scientists". When they finally stopped laughing, Jim wiped the tears from his face.

"That was a welcome fiasco," he admitted. "I've been so depressed since last night."

"I know exactly how you feel," Rodney echoed. "It's as though you see someone drowning before your eyes and you can't swim."

"Damn it, we're not going to lose this one," Jim blurted out. "Bob's going to raise holy hell if they try to bring Amstel here. We are headed for a real battle."

In Jim Kulp's laboratory close by, Bill Michaelson was washing lab ware. Donna Beardsley was accomplishing one of the many routine repetitive chores which require time and effort, but not much thought. Bill was telling Donna of his troubles with the Obstetrics and Gynecology Department.

"For some reason Dr. Krecke seems to have it in for me and he won't let up. I guess he's sore because he felt foolish in front of the nurses, house staff and students, at a time he was trying to make me look stupid." He told Donna of the delivery in which he'd almost made the diagnosis of a hand delivery before Krecke did. "I certainly would not be dumb enough to antagonize him purposely. It just happened. He has made me lose my cool and occasionally challenge him. I think house staff may have too much influence on student grades anyway."

"Why don't' you talk to Jake Bourne? He's in charge of the teaching in his department, isn't he?" Donna asked.

"Yeah, but I don't quite know what to say. Students are supposed to endure some pressure from the house staff, but I believe Krecke is out to flunk me. I really think he hates me. If I told Dr. Bourne that, he'd think I was paranoid. As it is, I think Krecke is nuts."

"You may well be right," mused Donna.

"Why do you think that? Did Andy have trouble with him?"

Donna, who had been lost in thought, turned toward Bill and said a little too emphatically not to raise his suspicions, "No. It's just some things I've heard."

"What things?"

"I'd rather not say, Bill, but keep your eyes open and be really careful in your dealings with him."

"Krecke is in line to be chief resident in OB. We can't avoid him and next week he'll quiz us orally and determine our grades for the session. I'm sure he'll flunk me if he can."

"Now you're being foolish. If you have performed reasonably well and your written final exam in OB is passing, he'll not be able to flunk you."

"That's true, but a lousy grade won't help me in getting a good internship. Maybe I ought to go and talk with him and try to get things on a better footing. After all, I won't have to deal with him forever, and I can swallow my pride long enough to get him off my back."

"That sounds sensible, but be careful," warned Donna.

Later that morning, Bill found Dr. Krecke on the obstetrics ward and asked to speak with him alone. The resident took him to his small office, closed the door and asked, with no trace of friendliness, what Bill wanted.

"I realize that somehow I have antagonized you Bill began.

Krecke interrupted, "Assuming that's true, of what consequence is it?"

Bill was stymied by Krecke's reply. After a moment's thought. he decided to be open and direct with the resident. "I think you have not been fair with me."

"In what way?"

"I get more than my share of routine work and am in on fewer of the interesting and instructional cases."

"Can you document that charge?" There were faint traces of a smile around Krecke's mouth.

"Of course not, but…"

"Then don't waste my time with your nonsensical accusations." Krecke was now angry but in control. "Whether I like you or not is of no consequence," he went on. "Aside from patient care, I'm here to teach and evaluate the students on my service, and that I do. If you are competent, you'll have no problem. If you're not you had better become competent and not waste my time with foolish matters." He stood up signaling the discussion was at an end.

Bill felt thoroughly helpless and dejected. He felt certain his attempt to set things right with Krecke had failed and confirmed his feelings that the man was out to hurt his reputation as a student. He was about to leave when a thought struck him and he turned and asked, "What can I do to improve my standing with you?"

For the first time Krecke smiled. "I'll tell you, but don't repeat it, cause I'll deny it. You can flunk out of school!"

Bill stood staring at Krecke, shocked at his words. The smile vanished from the doctor's face. "It's smart asses like you who drag medicine down to the level of a trade. This noble profession is tottering, subject to more and more governmental intervention; more liberals proposing health care programs for the undeserving; more inferior students getting aid to send them through medical school..." He went on in this vein, becoming more and more agitated and his arguments harder and harder to follow until they seemed irrational to Bill who remained still and silent. Krecke wound down slowly like a mechanical doll, When he had finally finished he stood for several seconds, trance-like, before he again took notice of Bill. As if nothing had happened he calmly and unemotionally asked, "Is there anything further I can do for you?"

Bill quickly excused himself and left the office. He's nuts, he thought, what do I do now? He'd confide in Donna and Andy and get some advice. This man was sick mentally. Was he seriously so or just over tired and this outburst of a temporary condition? Why the hell didn't his course in psychiatry give him some useful information instead of the thoroughly confused mass of information they tried to pass off as scientific? Whatever Krecke's problem it presented Bill with a more immediate one: that of passing Obstetrics and maintaining his scholarship support.

Jim Kulp was appalled at the manner in which the meeting was being conducted. Owing to an emergency, John Block could not attend and Charlie Evans was acting as chairman. Everyone, with the possible exception of Harry Tatum for whom these confrontations were being conducted, was minimizing the importance of the errors and distortions which appeared in Amstel's scientific publications. When Jim's turn to question Amstel came, he wisely avoided the small errors and emphasized the control data for the male and female mouse studies. He regretted John Block's absence when Amstel freely admitted that the data were from the same group of mice and, therefore, were inappropriate for one of the studies. He was unsure which. Amstel again insisted he had done the proper controls and was mystified as to why the proper controls had not been published. He passed the mistake off as a careless error. Dick Shane kept insisting that none of these insignificant errors changed the conclusions he'd drawn.

Jim decided to try another tack entirely. "Dr. Amstel," he asked, "you wish to be head of this Pharmacology Department. You know how we feel. Suppose you were our leader in our present position in this situation. How would you, as an administrator, handle this?" Jim sat back for the first time feeling as if he had really asked a good question. Amstel's administrative abilities had been touted by the Search Committee—let's see how he handles this one. He, Amstel, would have to explain just how he would lead a group of "fastidious scientists" for whom he seemed to have little respect, to accept sloppy science. Before Amstel could answer, the chairman broke in.

"I don't consider that a proper question for these proceedings."

"Why not? He wants to lead our department. Surely it's pertinent," Jim insisted.

"That has nothing to do with Dr. Amstel's publications which we are here to discuss," Dick Shane broke in.

Jim was thoroughly frustrated; but at least he had made sure that a serious error, that of the control data mix-up, had not been overlooked. Harry Tatum had specifically said he would have to have that error satisfactorily explained before he could vote to bring Amstel to Wilder. It had not been. It was also painfully clear that all the committee except Jim and possibly Harry Tatum were sympathetic toward Amstel. Whether or not that sympathy, which Jim himself had previously felt, would extend to voting to bring him to Wilder he did not know.

The meeting finished and Jim returned to the Pharmacology Department. He was met by an anxious group wanting to know how the session had gone. They were not at all surprised by Jim's description.

"What do we do now?" Jim asked.

"Have you given Block my message?" Bob Mettlar asked.

"I didn't get the chance. He wasn't there."

"Be certain that you do, Jim."

Jim hoped to bring the views of the department and the Search Committee closer together. He considered the men with whom he was dealing to be basically reasonable. He believed the departmental position, based as it was on Amstel's own written record, to be logical and unemotional. If looked at logically and unemotionally the Search Committee and the department would have to come to agree. Delivering Bob Mettlar's warning to go as high as the governor and the legislature would not foster an atmosphere of calm deliberation. He would hold his message as long as was possible.

Jim's membership in both camps was beginning to distress him. Though his sympathies were mainly with the department he had to consider both positions since he represented both sides. He came to realize that his actions about which he had at first felt quite virtuous, were being dictated for him by circumstance. He could behave in no other manner. He felt trapped. Now things were beginning to get difficult. He was making a decision to ignore the wishes, at least temporarily, of his former chief, Professor Mettlar. His respect for the man made him uncomfortable in doing so. Especially since it required that he consider his judgment in this matter superior to Bob's. He was unused to this degree of self-confidence and it did not materialize easily.

Amstel's visit ended without further excitement. His entire visit was anticlimactic, far worse in the anticipation than in the reality. The man's carefree attitude, which made the confrontations much less traumatic than they might have been and were appreciated from that aspect, now began to frighten the department. How could a scientist make so light of science? Was he sick? What explanation could fit his behavior?

To the committee, the department's attitude seemed rigid. They could not understand why an explanation of the errors and ambiguities in his published works would not suffice to make him an acceptable candidate to lead them. Granted his scientific image was somewhat tarnished, but their opinion of the department was not the highest, and they were too unfeeling to realize their actions made this quite apparent. Under these circumstances, trying to bring the two groups together to reach a settlement acceptable to both was probably unrealistic. Yet, such a meeting was scheduled as Jim was bound to try.

SUMMER

Jake Bourne was lecturing to the entire third-year class. The Thursday noon lecture period was one of two, hour long, lectures which were set aside weekly for the entire class to attend no matter to which clinical clerkship the students were assigned. The schedule was determined a year in advance and each of the major clinical departments was given some time. Obstetrics and gynecology were given five such lectures and three of these were given by Jake. His lectures were well attended by students, house staff, nurses and even occasional attending physicians, not so much because they were truly good, but because they were also entertaining. Jake had the reputation for tormenting the third year students. He would stop his lecture at any point and ask the students questions. His quick wit and sharp tongue would play havoc with the ego of any unprepared student.

Today, he was lecturing on the hormonal changes which take place during the menstrual cycle and during pregnancy. There are several hormones involved and their actions on the ovaries, uterus and other organs at various times during the cycle are complex and require lots of effort to memorize, let alone understand. After he had completed an explanation of a rather involved diagram he had constructed during his lecture, he stopped, looked at his list of students and asked, Is Dr. Michaelson present?" Bill raised his hand. "Please come to the blackboard. Doctor." Bill walked down the isle and up onto the platform where Jake stood.

"Now Dr. Michaelson, I presume you were paying attention and understood the interrelationships I just pointed out." He was about to continue his question when Bill interrupted.

"Sir, I was paying attention, but I did not understand the relationships." Jake stared at Bill for several seconds. "I'll grant this is complicated." Much to his audience's surprise, he refrained from chiding Bill and went through the lengthy explanation a second time. When he'd finished he asked, "Now do you understand?"

"No!" Bill answered. There was a noticeable decrease in sound in the lecture hall. Jake stared at Bill for some time and then again went through the explanation, this time in a slow and deliberate manner. When he'd finished, he said forcefully, "Now Goddamn it, do you understand?"

Bill was rattled. He could hear his answer as though he were a third party observing the scene. "No Goddamn it, I don't."

An absolute silence pervaded the room. Bill thought What have I done? Students don't swear at Professors. The silence continued. Jake stood staring at Bill who stared back not knowing what else to do. Slowly, a smile broke over Jake's face. He walked over to Bill, placed his hand on his shoulder, and led him off the lectern and up the aisle toward his seat. "You go home and sleep on it. Maybe it will come to you," he said. He returned to the lectern and continued as though nothing had happened.

His stock had definitely risen among his classmates that day and he enjoyed the notoriety he was receiving. He hoped the incident would not cause him more trouble in passing the Obstetrics course. and he wondered whether Dr. Krecke had mentioned him to Jake Bourne. He guessed not since Jake had treated him in an uncharacteristic manner. Perhaps no one had ever fought back when bullied by Bourne and he, Bourne, respected and even sought signs of courage in his students. After all Jake would not know that Bill's outburst was the response of a completely agitated student rather than a brave one. Whatever the reasons for Jake's forbearance, Bill was encouraged to turn to him for help should he need it in the future.

Dick Shane and John Block met in John's office. Their first meeting since Amstel's visit, they were planning their strategy.

"What did you think of his visit?" Shane asked.

"Remarkable, the way he handled himself under those circumstances. He is one cool customer."

"Do you think he will make a good chairman?"

"I think he'd be an excellent chairman in an administrative sense. I wouldn't hire him as a lab technician," John smiled as he said that.

"Do you think the Pharmacology Department has a legitimate gripe?"

"In theory, yes. In reality, he's our only candidate. From my perspective, his attributes outweigh his foibles. Dean Mackenzie wants him. Most of the Search Committee want him. Only the department objects and it isn't their choice. We'll get him here yet. He wants to come despite the fuss."

"In this afternoon's meeting with the Pharmacology Department, what do we hope to accomplish?" Shane asked.

"If we can, we'd like to smooth over the differences and get them to accept Amstel as an administrative head. If we emphasize the administration angle, we might just swing it. The department has fared badly under Bob Mettlar's leadership. It's the smallest department in the Medical School. We can truthfully point out that Amstel would make the department grow, get them more space and personnel, and lessen their teaching load. It's obvious Amstel would place his efforts on teaching and administration rather than research. That might actually help research freeing the other members time for it."

"What do you think of their research?"

"There is no question that Bob Mettlar is good," John admitted. "He's a crazy son of a bitch as far as I am concerned, but he's internationally recognized as a very good researcher. Rodney Barret, too, has an excellent national image. The rest are not well known. Dean Mackenzie tends to be critical of their teaching, but that's because they are conscientious teachers and require and get much from the students. The complaining types cry on the Dean's shoulder and he listens. Frankly, from observing their students in third and fourth year, I think they do one of the best jobs of all the Basic Sciences.

"Bob wouldn't have a graduate student program in Pharmacology. He prefers to train post doctorate students with degrees in biochemistry, organic chemistry or medicine. He may have a point. At any rate, with no graduate students to do their teaching for them, his faculty does it all. The students who have the stuff come to us well trained in the use of drugs. The poor ones who do slip by, do so at the Dean's insistence."

"In view of what you've just said and those ambiguities in Amstel's papers. why don't we seriously consider Rodney Barret as head?"

"We've gone too far with Amstel despite a note I received from him generously relieving our committee of any responsibility to him. More important, however, is the fact that Frank Mackenzie doesn't want Rodney."

"Why not?"

"I don't know, but he let me know in no uncertain terms. It's Amstel or we begin all over again, and I'm not for that."

When they met that afternoon, there was definite coolness despite the summer's heat. The two groups sat apart with few smiles and little cordial conversation. John Block reviewed the happenings which had brought them to this meeting. When he had finished and asked, "any questions?", Bob Mettlar rose.

Bob cleared his throat and looking at the ceiling said, "Our objections to Dr. Amstel are based primarily on his published works, the shortcomings of which cannot be explained away. In addition, however, his performance, on this last visit, no matter how admirable from the point of trying to put us at our ease, was truly remarkable. How a man could still want to come to a department which does not respect his work, is incomprehensible."

"Bob," John interrupted, "assuming for the moment that he is not a first class investigator, don't you think he would make a good administrator?"

"I don't care if he is the world's best administrator. We are not asking him here to be an assistant Dean. How can you ask someone to head a scientific department who has demonstrated such disrespect for science?"

Shane spoke up., "That's merely your opinion."

"Certainly, it is my opinion and the opinion of any reasonably intelligent person who reads those papers," Bob countered.

Shane bristled. "We contacted several people of national stature at his institution. They all said he was a capable and competent investigator."

"Then they have not read his work or they are not very critical," Mettlar insisted.

John Block interrupted, "Gentlemen, this is getting us nowhere. Bob, are you speaking for the entire department or are those only your views you've expressed?"

Rodney Barret answered. "He speaks for all of us, John." The other departmental members signaled assent.

"Then Amstel's visit did nothing to change your minds?"

"How could it?" asked Rodney.

"You're too damned rigid!" said an exasperated Shane.

"What do you expect from us, Dick?" Jim Kulp asked. "Amstel appears to despise what most of us has chosen as a way of life. Why should we want him to lead us?"

"You're overdramatizing, Jim," Shane replied.

"The hell I am!"

"Gentleman," Block broke in again. Let's keep this discussion free of emotion. You realize the choice of a head is the Search Committee's and not the Department's prerogative."

Rodney answered, "We realize that, John. We're only requesting that you not offer the job to Amstel for obvious reasons. If you've already offered him the job, say so. We won't be happy about it, but speaking for myself, I'd understand. If you haven't, please don't."

"We haven't offered him the job," John flatly stated. There was silence. "It appears that nothing this committee can say will alter your position?" he asked.

The department communicated their universal agreement.

"Well, gentlemen, this meeting is over. We'll do what we have to do and see how it all comes out."

Bob Mettlar rose and informed the Search Committee of his intentions to go as high as the governor to prevent their bringing in Amstel as head. The committee was truly shocked and several members were obviously furious, but Bob, seemingly unaware, left the room before their fury could be vented on him.

"That man is insane!" said John Block.

"The hell he is," countered Jim Kulp.

"I say he is," repeated John.

"I say he isn't," insisted Jim.

"I guess it boils down to which of you is the better clinician," cut in Rodney Barret trying to inject some levity into a tense situation, It was funny in view of the fact that John Block was the acting head of Medicine and Jim's clinical experience had been limited to his medical school curriculum. No one even noticed.

Clearly, the divergent points of view had completely polarized and Jim sided with his department. Again John Block announced the termination of the joint meeting, but asked the Search Committee members to stay for further deliberations. When the departmental members left, Jim Kulp sat surrounded by empty chairs. His geographical estrangement was accompanied by a psychological estrangement, and John Block pointedly ignored him as he spoke to the committee.

"I will transmit your desires to Dean Mackenzie as soon as possible. How many vote to bring Sidney Amstel here as departmental chairman?" All hands went up except for Jim's. Jim looked at Harry Tatum and thought, Why did you put us through those confrontations? Amstel didn't answer your concerns, yet you're voting to bring him here anyway. He felt alone and confused.

Discouraged, Marie Barret had not felt well for ages. Though for a time, she thought she was improving, now she felt she was losing ground. She requested an office visit with Peter Markley rather than the brief shoulder pat, smile and "uh-huh" she received from him on his occasional visits to the unit while she was dialyzing. Again she sat in his examining table in the scanty paper examining robe designed poorly to save one's dignity and not at all one's body heat. She wondered just how much longer she would have to endure the nausea and ever present headache she seemed to have. The lethargy, that was the worst part, no desire to do anything, not even things which had been important to her only eight months ago. Her visits to the dialysis unit were now made with mixed feelings. One side of her was interested in her new friends, strongly linked by sharing a dependence upon life-sustaining equipment, and part of her despised the dependence upon this mass of blood-filled tubing, dials and alarms. She had been an alert and busy person contrasted with the uncaring lethargy in which she was being enveloped. Though a paradox, she cared.

Peter entered the room and quickly accomplished his physical examination and read her chart for several minutes before he turned and faced her. "Well, Marie what can I do for you.?"

"Peter, I do not feel I'm making any progress. Am I getting any worse?"

Peter looked directly at Marie for several seconds before he spoke. "I can't detect any signs of deterioration in your physical or laboratory studies. Your blood pressure is up a bit more than I would like to see. I'll adjust your medication. Precisely why do you ask?"

"I'm discouraged. I don't ever seem to feel well anymore. I'm losing interest in almost everything, perhaps life itself. I go from treatment to treatment, and if anything I feel worse. Isn't there something we can do to improve the situation?"

"Your adjustment to this situation may be the basis of your trouble."

"How do you mean?"

"Tell me, Marie, how do you perceive your present over all problem?"

"I'm not sure I understand your question?"

"How would you describe your medical problem?"

Marie thought for a few moments. "I'm crippled by the loss of kidney function. I'm at the mercy of a relatively new and as yet unperfected technology. I am kept alive but not well. Is that what you mean?"

"Yes, that is what I was getting at. Your perception is accurate as far as it goes. You have not yet completely come to terms with the situation. Some patients do well in your situation and others do not. I'm not really sure just why this is, whether it is physiological or psychological. I would have predicted you would do well. Your faith, your family, your energy, your drive, I felt would sustain you."

"That's just the problem, the drive and interest are lacking. I've never lacked them before. I feel guilty precisely because of that lack."

Peter laughed. "Your loss of drive and energy are completely understandable. You can't be expected to keep going at the old pace, but that doesn't mean you are through. Accept some limitations and perform within them. How much help do you have at home?"

"The kids help some. Rodney helps more now, but I manage. It's just not the fun it used to be.."

Peter's face showed surprise. "You mean you don't have live-in help?"

"A maid comes in twice a week."

"Who does the cooking?"

"I do."

"Who car pools the kids?"

"I do some, and I have a babysitter for my dialysis days."

"Good Lord, Marie, you do a lot, too much."

"But it is so much less than I used to do."

Peter realized that Marie judged herself by a very high standard and that what he would perceive as a minor restriction Marie would consider major.

"In view of all you are doing, I think your physiological adjustment is good, very good indeed. If you were to rest more and spare yourself you might feel better. Damn it, get more help."

"I like to do things my own way, I don't like help. Besides, frankly, we can't afford it. This illness is a real drain on our finances."

"I know," he nodded.

"Aren't there some pills you can give me to help me feel more my old self? I used to enjoy sex. I don't any more."

"If you spared yourself, you might." Peter wondered if this was at the heart of Marie's poor adjustment. He talked with Linda about every patient and Linda was a good observer, yet she had said little of Marie. Had she missed seeing her obvious unhappiness? He couldn't believe that.

"There aren't any magic potions which make up for a loss of kidney function except perhaps a transplant and that's too new to evaluate yet. How is the shunt doing?"

"It clogs occasionally, but Linda is a whiz at unstopping it The wound infection is minimal. Right now it's in good shape. I've even learned how to hide it for formal occasions."

She can't be too badly off if she attends formal occasions, he thought. He smiled.

"Marie, now that we've had this talk, I hope you will somehow get more help and more rest. I'll talk with Rodney about it."

"I wish you wouldn't."

"Why? He should be supportive."

"I know, but he's having a rough time right now with the departmental search going on."

"There is always some reason you give to spare Rodney at your own expense. For once, listen to me. Let's make Rodney more responsible to your problem. Don't shut him out trying to spare him. I presume he wants to help all he can?"

"I'm not sure." Marie sounded truly uncertain and very unhappy. This was the first time Peter had heard her voice any doubts about her precious Rodney. He was quite aware of the havoc Marie's condition could play in family adjustments. Peter was silent hoping to further draw out her real feelings.

"Early next week the Executive Committee will meet to consider, among other things, the Pharmacology appointment," announced Dean Mackenzie in his office with a summoned Jim Kulp. "I want you to represent the Pharmacology Department."

"But Tony Lewis is acting head. Shouldn't he?"

"Tony will be away on vacation. You'll be the one."

Frank Mackenzie's Executive Committee, made up of all the departmental chairmen, was in the final analysis, purely advisory. With Tony away, Frank was afraid Bob Mettlar might represent the department, and he did not want that. He felt Jim Kulp would be easier to control.

"Dean Mackenzie, can I speak frankly with you?"

"Damn it, Jim, I don't want to hear anything more about those publications. All I get is a rehash."

Jim had learned that "rehash" meant to the Dean anything he chose not to hear.

"Sir, I do not want to discuss that situation with you. I only want to ask you some questions about the Executive Committee meeting since I have never attended one before."

Frank Mackenzie's attitude toward Jim changed. He'd been cool and business like, but once he realized Jim was not going to argue, he became much friendlier.

"What would you like to know?"

"Well, how will the meeting proceed? The Search Committee wants Amstel. They will recommend him to the Executive Committee. How will I voice my objections?"

"John Block will present the majority opinion to the Executive Committee. You, then, will have the chance to present the minority opinion. Then the departmental chairman will have a chance to ask the Search Committee any questions they choose. Then the Search Committee will leave and the Executive Committee members will discuss and vote on the Search Committee recommendations.'

"You want me to stay and represent the department for that?"

"Absolutely."

Jim was surprised. Though someone had to represent the department it offended his sense of fair play to think he'd be able to stay on after the rest of the Search Committee had been dismissed. He could, then, continue to try and influence the Executive Committee. He guessed it was probably Frank Mackenzie's fear of having Bob Mettlar present that dictated this circumstance. He would make the most of it. It wasn't his doing.

"What day is the meeting, sir?"

The Dean consulted his calendar. "Monday afternoon at two," he answered. "You should have your minority report in a written form and hand it in at that time."

"For some reason, John Block has told me not to talk with anyone about our vote yesterday. In fact he's told me not to talk with anyone in the department until after the Executive Committee meeting. Do you agree with that?"

"That does seem a bit extreme, but in view of the emotions this search seems to have stirred up, perhaps it's best."

"Will you tell the department I'll represent them at the meeting if I'm not to talk with them?"

"For goodness sake, Jim, don't be so literal. Go tell them yourself. Just don't discuss any thing you shouldn't. I trust your judgment."

"Others don't. John told me to stay away from the department entirely."

"Well I'm telling you to go there now. Tell Bob or Rodney or even the departmental secretary what's up, and then go home and write your report and be here Monday at two."

"May I use your secretary to type it?"

Dean Mackenzie looked bored and annoyed. "Bring your report to my secretary early Monday morning and she'll type it for you. Just don't write a book!"

"I could, you know," Jim grinned.

"Don't!" the dean said without a smile.

To avoid future difficulties Jim went straight to his home. He telephoned the department and informed Donna and the departmental secretary that he would not be in and to refer any calls to his home. He sat at his desk to compose his minority report. Janet and his youngest offspring were playing nearby and the occasional shrieks and laughter broke his attempts at concentration. He found himself annoyed with them for not realizing the seriousness of his endeavor and maintaining silence. He recognized his unreasonableness and wondered if he might transfer his literary efforts to his cottage at the lake. He rose from his desk and went to the porch where Janet and their youngest daughter were playing. The older children were at school. Janet was dressed casually in short shorts and one of his old shirts and looked her usual neat attractive self. As he viewed her long suntanned legs, other thoughts began to impinge on his cerebrum, and the idea of spending a monastic weekend was becoming less attractive. He was fighting an inner battle when a compromise solution to the situation occurred to him. If he could think of a diversion for the little one, he had some ideas for the big one and he could leave for the lake a reasoning man. He decided to put his plan into action.

Jake Bourne was making rounds on the Obstetrics-Gynecology ward. The Friday rounds were primarily for medical student teaching purposes and the patient's story was presented by the medical student to whom the patient was assigned. Jake's rounds, like his lectures, were attended by a few curious onlookers more interested in medical student baiting than in possibly witnessing an interesting case history. Since the Friday rounds were one chance for students to impress Jake, and since he invariably went down the left side of the ward first, each student, with the house staff's blessing, put the patient he or she knew best in one of the first beds on the left. The presentations usually took from ten to fifteen minutes, including Jake's quizzing, so that only four to six presentations could be accomplished in the one hour Jake assigned to his student rounds.

Among the first patients on the left was one Bill Michaelson had "worked up" thoroughly. This meant he had done her complete history and physical examination when she had appeared on the service and had followed her case daily since. Cases which were on the service when a new class of students arrived were assigned, but seldom evoked the interest or effort the students expended on the "new" patient they had "worked up" themselves. These patients beds were rolled to the right side of the ward for Friday rounds.

The student presenters were under pressure to do well as these rounds were thought to be responsible for a large portion of their grade on the service.

For reasons that no one has yet explained, this particular Friday Jake decided to go down the right side of the ward. This simple change produced an outpouring of adrenaline in the bodies of students with patients on the right which was pitiful to behold. Fred Stryker had the patient in the first bed on the right. He was a good student whose clinical presentations had always been competent. Today he was caught so completely by surprise that the little he did know about the patient went completely from his head. He looked deathly pale and he stammered. It took a supposedly surreptitious glance at the name plate at the foot of the bed for him to recall even the patient's name. In as much as these presentations were to be given without the aid of notes, his performance was unusually poor. If Jake was aware of the stir he had caused by his unhappy change of routine, he did not so indicate in any way. His questioning was unsympathetic and his utter dissatisfaction with Fred's performance was obvious.

When Fred's ordeal was over, Jake turned his attention to the second patient on the right. She was assigned to Joan Wentworth, daughter of an anatomy professor and an excellent student. While Fred Stryker was muddling through his presentation, Joan had managed to review this second patient's history, physical, and hospital course from notes she had taken from the patient's chart and kept in a small notebook in her pocket. All students carried such notebooks, and it was usual to refer to them except at the time of presentations to Jake. Fred's fiasco allowed others the luxury of slipping to the rear of the assembled onlookers and quickly reviewing this source of information. A patient of Bill Michaelson's was in the fourth bed on the right and he, too, was glancing at his notes.

When Joan had finished a relatively good presentation and had fielded Jake's questions, he went on to the third patient,. No student came forth to present.

"Whose patient is this?" Jake asked.

No one answered. Jake called Dr. Krecke who was standing in the nurse's station. "Who is assigned to this patient?" he repeated.

Krecke sauntered leisurely down the ward to where the group was standing. He looked in the bed. "Mrs. Murray came in last night. She was assigned to Michaelson."

Bill was dumbfounded, He could feel his heart racing for the second time during these rounds. It had just slowed down from his realization of having to present Mrs. Ford in the fourth bed of whom he was relatively unfamiliar.

"Well, Bill, tell us about her," Jake demanded.

"I can't"

"How so?" Jake seemed unusually calm under the circumstances.

"To be honest, Dr. Bourne, this is the first time I have laid eyes on her. I didn't realize she was my patient."

Jake turned to Krecke. "What's the foul-up here?"

"I don't know, Jake. I told Bill Mrs. Murray was coming in last night."

"When did you tell him?"

"Before the ten o'clock dead line as in our policy," Krecke answered.

"What about that, Bill?" Jake was calm but unsmiling.

Bill realized it was his word against Krecke's. He had no recollection of even talking with Krecke since his distressing interview the previous week.

"I don't know what to say Dr. Bourne. I cannot remember Dr. Krecke assigning Mrs. Murray to me. In fact, Don Peck was supposed to be next in rotation for a new patient. Isn't that so Fred?" He asked Fred Stryker who acted as student coordinator.

Fred who had barely recovered from his harrowing presentation, said, "Don is in the infirmary. He went in last night." A silence followed.

Jake's voice cut in. "Let's get on with it. Whose is the next patient?"

"Mine," gulped Bill.

Jake looked annoyed. "Go ahead," he said without enthusiasm. Bill gave a good presentation considering he had just reviewed the case from reading his notebook in the back row. His patient had been delivered of a normal baby and hemorrhaged following the birth. They had been unable to stop the bleeding by the conservative method packing the uterus and had to resort to an emergency hysterectomy in which Mrs. Ford lost her uterus and the ability to reproduce, but not her life or her baby. When Bill had finished, Jake hypothesized a somewhat similar situation in which a patient was hemorrhaging profusely from her vaginal orifice following a delivery.

"How would you distinguish between a torn uterus and uterine atony (a condition in which the uterus stays flaccid instead of contracting as it normally does after a birth)?"he asked. He ignored Bill and instead pointed from one to the other of the present medical students. None answered. It wasn't in their textbook. He looked disgusted and finally his eyes met Bill's. "Do you know?" he asked.

Bill was not aware of this particular differential diagnosis from his reading, but simple logic suggested an answer. "A hand on her abdomen would tell you," he said.

Jake suddenly beamed. "Of course, tell them how," he indicated the other students.

"You wouldn't feel the uterus through the abdomen if it was atonic. A torn uterus would still contract, you'd feel it like we do after each delivery," Bill explained. He glanced at Krecke and noticed he was no longer smirking as he had been when accusing him of neglecting Mrs. Murray. That fact and Jake Bourne's change of manner toward him on answering his questions helped to restore his confidence after a disquieting morning. Still he was troubled. He knew Dr. Krecke was trying to discredit him. He knew he hadn't spoken to Krecke. He wouldn't be likely to forget a conversation with "that creep".

That afternoon, in Dr. Kulp's laboratory he told Donna about Krecke's lie to Jake Bourne about him. Donna seemed concerned as she always seemed to be when he described Krecke's machinations.

"I can't complain about him. No one would listen. He's been careful to limit his game to things I can't document. Besides, who wants the reputation for hurting one of the house staff even if he is crazy and unfair to students he dislikes?"

"But he should be stopped," Donna insisted.

"Not by me. The price is too high."

"When is your oral examination with him?"

"Monday morning."

"Will you be all alone with him?"

"I don't know,"

"Dr. Bourne knows you're not dumb. He'd be concerned if Krecke tried to flunk you."

"I guess you're right, Donna, but having him on my back makes me nervous. It's depressing knowing he's out to get me flunked out."

"I suppose so," said Donna who was thinking that she might not be able to stop Krecke entirely, but was certain she could get him to leave Bill alone.

What's Jim up to?" Rodney asked Donna when he had become aware of his absence. Jim was such a regular worker that any deviation from his routine was easily noticed.

"He called to say he's working on his report for the upcoming department's head meeting. He won't be back till sometime after that's over Monday afternoon."

"Thanks Donna." Rodney wondered how Jim would perform his duty as minority opinion wielder against the rest of the Search Committee. He knew that the committee would not change its opinion, but would Jim be able to convince the department heads that Amstel was not a fit leader? He decided to explore these thoughts with Bob Mettlar.

That same evening Bill Michaelson had a date with Marian Marsh. Marian had transferred to Wilder at the end of the semester but, despite her attraction for him, he had seen little of her since their tour of the laboratory. His spare time was limited, and her beauty and personality made her popular and unavailable. Donna had encouraged Bill to see her and, liking Bill, had wanted Marian to like him too. Marian, though friendly, had remained cool. Bill arrived at her dormitory early in the evening. As he walked from his boarding house this warm summer evening he wondered why he was doing this. Though strongly attracted to Marian, he did not feel she was attracted to him. When she had not yet transferred to Wilder, he'd felt he had a chance with her, but now that she was here, the competition was fierce and Bill didn't have the stomach for it. He had made this date only at Donna's insistence.

Bill felt his lack of finances keenly. On the one hand he was fiercely independent, and if he needed a fancy car, expensive clothes, and the like to get a girl, he didn't want her. Yet his lack of wherewithal to date in the grand manner disturbed him. Consequently he tended to avoid Marian. Her response to this avoidance was coolness since she interpreted it as a lack of interest on his part. She liked Bill. His serious and intense nature in regard to his work intrigued her. She was pleased to be going out with him though she suspected Donna had encouraged the date. She was so popular and didn't need dates, and she knew Donna knew this, so she suspected her of serious matchmaking.

They greeted each other in a perfunctory, wary manner, each holding back lest the ether consider the other too eager. They agreed to walk into town for supper in a local bistro. They sat in a booth in the mainstream of the restaurant where several of the passing customers recognized Marian and stopped for a few words. None of Bill's acquaintances passed, and his feeling s of estrangement grew. Their conversation was strained and he again wondered why he had let Donna talk him into this. Neither found talking to the other easy as they had in their first encounters. Each held back feeling the other was not really interested. He became more and more uncomfortable as the meal progressed and felt the need for some athletic type of activity to relieve the tension in his stomach, He, therefore, suggested a brisk walk when they had finished dinner. Marian agreed and they set off walking down one of the quiet tree-lined streets. Neither spoke but concentrated on the exercise. Soon they arrived at the entrance to the Wilder University golf course. The evening was a beautiful one. A bright moon was rising to supplant the setting sun and it illuminated the country side to the degree that to their dark adapting eyes it was nearly as bright as day. The temperature was on the warm side, but a gentle breeze prevented it from being uncomfortable. As they were crossing an empty concrete parking lot Bill stopped and turned to Marian and asked, "Do you dance?"

"Yes," she replied.

He stood erect, held up his arms, and began to whistle a Strauss waltz.

With little hesitation, Marian stepped towards him, clasped his hands and off they went cavorting around the parking lot. With no one watching neither was the least bit inhibited and they danced to any tune either or both of them could whistle or hum. The evening was so beautiful that they imagined themselves the Astaire and Rogers of Wilder University, and danced for well over an hour. For both of them it was a delightful, exhilarating, spontaneous experience. They felt right; and generating the music from within, it was easy to keep music and movement synchronized. Their efforts warmed them and they decided to go for a swim in the lake on the golf course. As it was now late and no one was around, they shed their clothes and entered the water which was comfortably cool. They swam across the lake and back without saying a word. Bill self-consciously avoided looking at Marian and found the entire experience so beautiful that despite their nakedness he was not conscious of sexual desire. When they had reached a standing depth, Marian lost her footing and fell back into the water. She laughed and held her hand out to Bill for support. He took it, and they walked hand in hand up the bank. At the water's edge, without words, they turned and embraced. Her warm body pressed against did arouse him but it seemed so natural, so unstrained. They found a comfortable mossy area and made love.

When they had finished, he lay on his back looking at the stars with Marian nestled in the crook of his arm, his mind racing, his mood soaring. That this desirable girl cared for him, that he had made love to her—so naturally, so easily—was astounding The act itself, the coupling, the release, by themselves though sweet and exciting were really not that much If he'd believed all he'd read and heard, rockets should have fired, roller coasters should have traversed the moon, but nothing of the sort happened. His feelings were of relief and gratitude. Relief that he had finally had intercourse and gratitude that he had not made a fool of himself. Most of all he felt a closeness to this girl at his side he had never felt for another human being. She really seemed to care for him. That night, Bill lost his heart and virginity at one and the same time.

Monday afternoon the meeting of the Executive Committee was called to order by Dean Mackenzie.

"Ladies and Gentlemen, we are here, primarily to hear the report of the Pharmacology Search Committee. As you are undoubtedly aware, this particular search has not gone smoothly. The department has chosen to make its objections to the prime candidate known, and this afternoon you will have a chance to hear from the committee and a departmental representative. With your permission we will dispense with the usual formalities of minutes of the previous meeting and get down to business."

A murmur of assent greeted the Dean's questioning glances towards his various department heads who were seated at a long rectangular table in the Wilder General Hospital's board room where such meetings took place.

"Before turning over the floor to Dr. Shane for the Search Committee, I want to read to you a letter I received from the Pharmacology Department last week. It is addressed to you, the 'Advisory Committee of the Medical Faculty'. It goes as follows:

Gentlemen:

It is our understanding that a report from the Pharmacology Search Committee relative to the possible appointment of Dr. Sidney B. Amstel as chairman of our department will be presented to the Advisory Committee meeting. Although we have no knowledge of this report, we wish to make known our thoughts in regard to this matter known to you.

At the time the committee informed us that Dr. Amstel was a leading candidate for this position, in an honest effort to become better acquainted with his research, we read some of his recent papers. As a result

271

of these reviews of Dr. Amstels publications, it became a unanimous opinion of this department that they revealed an unacceptable degree of carelessness, obscurities and inaccuracies. These findings were immediately discussed in detail with the Search Committee.

At the committees request upon the specific desires of Dr. Amstel at the time of his last visit, members of the department were put into the embarrassing situation of having to point out these deficiencies to him. During these discussions, he freely admitted the deficiencies; but made light of them.

In view of this, it is the feeling of this department that Dr. Amstel's attitudes and standards toward science are below the level that this department, this medical school and this university are striving to maintain. In addition, it seemed unwise to bring to a department a chairman who has been fully apprised of the opinions that his faculty members hold concerning his scientific stature.

Finally, the effectiveness of a department in which a chairman is appointed under these circumstances would be seriously jeopardized.

"This letter is signed by all the members of the department with the exception of Dr. Kulp who is on the Search Committee."

"Why didn't he sign it?" asked Jake Bourne. Dean Mackenzie nodded to Jim.

"I didn't know they'd written such a letter until Dean Mackenzie just read it, but I would have signed it," Jim announced.

Jake looked puzzled. "Don't you talk to your department?" he asked.

"Since last Thursday, Dr. Block forbade me to."

Jake looked astounded. "Forbade you to?"

Dean Mackenzie interrupted. "You'll undoubtedly hear all the gory details before we're through, Jake. Let's go on. Dr. Shane will you give the majority report now?" He emphasized the word "majority".

Dick Shane rose from his chair and walked to the end of the long table. It was obvious he was nervous and exceedingly grim.

"Let me begin by stating that the Search Committee reaffirms its recommendation of Dr. Sidney B. Amstel for your consideration for the Chairmanship of the Pharmacology Department. The committee voted five to one for him, and you will undoubtedly be hearing a minority report from Dr. Kulp." He glanced unhappily in Jim's direction.

"This selection is important because it is the first in a series which must be made. It will, therefore, serve as a measure for future selections and by his seniority this chairman, will have an important voice in the faculty councils of this medical school. At the same time the committee is aware of limited space and monies to help attract a first-class candidate...not to mention the presence in the department of the former chairman. Several chairs of Pharmacology are presently unfilled around the country. Frankly, gentleman, competition is great, and we don't have a great deal to offer." The sounds of muted conversation were again heard, and Dr. Shane cleared his throat and waited for silence before continuing.

"During these past nine months, we screened some ninety candidates. Twenty-three candidates from other schools were invited to be considered for the position. Five affirmative responses were received, and three visited the school. Two declined further interest. Despite this minimal interest, the majority of this committee believe this search has been accomplished with success as indicated in our recommendation. The one dissenting vote reflects the attitudes of the members of the Department of Pharmacology. I would like now to consider the objections of the department in our total appraisal of Dr. Amstel.

"To begin with, Dr. Amstel has a distinguished background. He has received honors and scholarships as you can see from his curriculum vitae, copies of which were supplied you. He is considered a competent scientist, Pharmacology's views not withstanding, by the dean of his medical school, his department head, and other world-renowned scientists at his present prestigious institution. He visited this school and at the time there was no objections voiced to his candidacy. Four of the committee members fully supported our recommendation to Dean Mackenzie that Dr. Amstel be offered the chair and the other two found this acceptable. The Dean, then, invited Dr. Amstel for a second visit with his wife. Days later, the committee learned that members of the Pharmacology Department had objections. We invited a representative to present the department's views. At this meeting the committee was informed of certain errors and ambiguities discovered in the last five publications which, in the opinion of the department, cast serious doubt on his scientific competence. The

Search Committee considered these and following prolonged deliberation elected to inform Dr. Amstel that these questions had been raised in order to seek his answers. We met with the department to obtain the questions which were uppermost in their minds concerning the errors and ambiguities. We were informed by the department that there could not exist any possible explanation which could be acceptable to the department.

"The chairman of the Search Committee met with Dr. Amstel prior to his scheduled appointments. At that time, Dr. Amstel was informed about the complaint of the errors and ambiguities but their source was not revealed. Dr. Amstel requested the source so that he might face his accusers rather than act through an intermediary. He was provided that information and subsequently met with members of the department.

"Later, with the Search Committee, he declared that he considered the Search Committee relieved of all its responsibility to him. He further acknowledged the presence of computation errors. He was also disturbed by the points of ambiguity, but he stated unequivocally that the experiments had been performed as described and that any connotations to the contrary were unfounded. He could not understand the extreme reaction manifested by the department in response to the papers, a response which seemed to preclude discussion and clarification.

"Following this visit, the committee again met with the department to assess their views. In brief, nothing had occurred to change their views.

"In summary, we do not agree with the department's charge of scientific incompetence. Dr. Amstel has demonstrated mature judgment, articulateness, and dignity under extremely trying circumstances. These are qualities admirable in a departmental chairman. Finally, as a consequence of the invitation extended by this medical school to Dr. Amstel for a second visit with its attendant implications, the honor and integrity of the school may be jeopardized by any other decision."

During Shane's recital, Jim observed most of the department heads seemed bored or uninterested. They seldom looked at the speaker but sat quietly looking down at the table. Now it was his turn. He awaited Dean Mackenzie's introductory remarks and in view of the cordial terms on which they had parted prior to the weekend, he was entirely unprepared for the introduction which followed.

"Dr. Kulp will now present his minority report of this appalling situation. I hope he will be brief in his rehash. We have been embarrassed enough already by the inept manner in which this search has been conducted. Dr. Amstel would obviously make an excellent head so let's get on with it. Dr. Kulp give your report; but for pity's sake, make it brief!"

Jim rose and walked to the head of the table. The Dean glared at him. Most of the department heads looked uncomfortable, few looked at him. Only Dr. Fraser, of Surgery and Jake Bourne of Obstetrics and Gynecology looked him in the eye and appeared to be sympathetic. The Dean's words and manner, though disturbing, reminded Jim of his first experience on a locked psychiatry ward when he was a third year medical student. He had just entered the ward when a disturbed female patient berated him with obscenities and fanciful accusations. He was startled and embarrassed, but for the patient, not for himself. He'd had the same reaction to Dean Mackenzie's introduction.

As he began his report he concentrated on Fraser and Bourne.

"It is my duty to present you a dissenting view on Dr. Amstel. I do so with some sadness because I know him better than any of you since we came from the same school. I admit, that though I was not enthusiastic about choosing him as department head, it was not until I read his paper's, that I had serious objections to it. I will do my best to convince you that he should not be brought here as departmental chairman of Pharmacology. My objections are based on his own published work.

"His last five publications are the only one with which I am familiar, but these contain errors and inconsistencies which are alarming. A striking feature of these papers is that whenever the reader is presented enough data to check one item against another, some distortion becomes apparent. The committee states that these admitted distortions do not change the conclusions drawn in the papers. That may be true, but is there any reason to assume there are fewer distortions in the data the reader cannot check.

"In my position as a departmental member and a committee member, I have observed the actions of both. I am forced to conclude that the group that arrived at its decision with a minimum of emotional and inconsistent behavior ought to have arrived at the more valid conclusion.

"I am convinced that no department should be allowed to dictate who its departmental chairman should be. I cannot, however, interpret the actions of the Pharmacology Department in any way other than extreme concern for this school.

"As a Search Committee member, I feel guilty that the papers in question were not read prior to the candidates first visit to this campus. I do not feel I can accept the responsibility for the greatest mistake of all—that of offering Dr. Amstel this chair."

When he finished, the silence and seeming lack of attention paid to his presentation was a depressing anticlimax to his long weekend of preparation.

"Thank you for your minority report." The word "minority" was stressed this time by the Dean. "Are there any questions the advisory committee members would like to ask the Search Committee before we dismiss them?" the Dean asked.

"What's all this crap about Block forbidding Kulp to talk to his department until after this meeting?" Jake Bourne demanded.

John Block looked cool and fully in control as he answered Jake. The effort he was using to remain so would have been apparent only to those who knew him well.

"Dr. Kulp's responsibilities in this search have placed him in a peculiar position. I felt this minority report should be his and not the department's. I, therefore, suggested he avoid departmental members until after this meeting."

Suggested, my arse, thought Jake.

"If I understand this correctly, all the objections to this candidate spring from five scientific publications?" stated Dr. Fraser.

"Yes, sir," Jim answered.

"How were these chosen?" Fraser asked.

"They were his last five publications."

"What about his previous work?"

"I haven't read any of it," Jim answered.

"I can speak to that," John Block asserted. "If anything, his past work, which has been reviewed critically, does not show any apparent calculation errors and, if anything, presents data in amounts more than necessary to support his conclusions. There is another point I would like to make regarding these errors. When I was first made aware of this problem, I went to Professor Mary White to get an objective view. We read the papers together, and made some of the calculations, and we made some errors. Didn't we Mary?" John Block smiled at her.

"Yes we did, John," Mary smiled back. "But we didn't publish!" This brought laughter but the smile vanished from John's face.

"Any further questions of the committee?" the Dean asked. After an appropriate silence he added, "the committee is dismissed. Thank you,gentleman, for your time."

The Search Committee with the exception of Jim Kulp rose to go.

John Block seeing that Jim was still sitting approached him from behind and in a fatherly manner placed his hand on Jim's shoulder. "Come, Jim we've been dismissed," he explained.

Jim, trying unsuccessfully to hide his obvious pleasure, turned around and answered, "John, I now change hats and become my department's representative at Dean Mackenzie's insistence."

Disbelief appeared on John's face and was rapidly followed by a solemn mask through which Jim sensed pure hatred. For an instant, he felt some of the satisfaction that he had not derived from his earlier presentation to the group. John turned and with the rest of the Search Committee left the room. When they had gone, the Dean called for discussion. Alfred Crane rose to speak representing the Department of Medicine whose chief could not be present. He wrinkled his considerable brow in apparent deep thought.

"It is inconceivable to me," he began, "that we consider bringing Dr. Amstel in to head a department which feels about him the way in which this one does. All other considerations aside, it would be sheer folly. For this reason, I move that we table the recommendation of the Pharmacology Search Committee to offer Dr. Amstel this position." He sat down. Again there was silence.

The Dean looked around the table but no one had anything to say. "A motion has been made. Do I hear a second?"

"I second," Jake Bourne raised his hand.

"Is there discussion?" the Dean asked, but silence followed." A motion to table has been made and seconded. All those in favor say aye." There was a mumbling of ayes.

"Those opposed?" Silence followed. "The motion to table passes. I think you are making a mistake, but at least I know the sense of this advisory groups feelings in this matter."

The meeting was adjourned with the recognition that the group would meet again the following afternoon to take up some other matters which needed attention.

Jim was let down and disillusioned. His position had won out but not for the right reasons. Amstel, hopefully, would not be offered the chair. No one admitted Amstel wasn't a proper candidate. They just suggested he couldn't lead a pack of soreheads who didn't want him and that just was not the case. As he was leaving he came upon Mary White who said, "You did a fine job, Jim."

"Thanks, Mary, but I don't feel any satisfaction. I might as well have not been there."

"I don't believe that is so," Mary replied. "Just wait, Jim some day what you did will stand you in good stead." Jim was pleased to hear her remark, but as he was to say some decades later, "I'm still waiting."

Back in his office overlooking the city and the well-traveled river, Sidney Amstel wondered just how much he really wanted the position at Wilder. At this very moment he knew he was being considered by Dean Mackenzie's advisory committee. He didn't like to think of what might be going on. He was annoyed. After all, he was a good teacher and administrator. He liked preparing and giving lectures. He liked preparing courses and the work he did in his editorship. The day to day grind of research wasn't his bag. He found it boring. Results were seldom clear-cut, and you couldn't cut and prune as with lecture material. You were allowed license to make the lecture material understandable. In research, errors could be unearthed and thrown at you, just as had recently occurred.

He had acquitted himself well, he felt, on his recent visit. He knew a majority of the Search Committee were for him. Only the department seemed against him, and even they were friendly. He could not understand why the petty errors they had discovered had caused such a furor. Granted the papers weren't great, but he felt they fulfilled his obligation to publish. With the exception of Bob Mettlar he was probably better known than any of them. He was editor-in-chief of a prominent scientific journal which had grown in thickness since he had taken over the editorship. He had written textbooks. It was unfair that publication, which to him was a minor function, seemed to carry so much weight. Jim Kulp had said if he had never published anything he would be for him. It was the poor publications to which Jim had objected. He should never have dashed off those papers. Others had noticed them, too, and they had come back to haunt him.

He hadn't said anything to Barbara about the confrontations he had undergone on the visit. They had gone smoothly. The worst, the one with Mettlar, Barret and Kulp hadn't really been too bad., though he did not feel he had made much of a dent in the position of the Pharmacology department. They seemed awfully rigid in their attitudes. Too rigid for their own good. It was obvious they needed someone with his abilities to build up the department.

Would they offer him the chairmanship? He felt they would, but he wasn't certain. Was there anything he could do? He thought, not, at this point.

His note to the committee absolving them of any responsibility to him subsequent to the confrontations was, he thought, a good touch. He felt he couldn't hold them to their verbal offer in a court of law anyway, so acting in what appeared to be a mature and reasonable manner could only help him. He did want to hear from them soon. Would he take the position if offered it? He really wasn't one hundred percent certain, but he desperately wanted the choice to be his. He wanted to show Barbara that offer whether he took it or not.

Jim returned to the department eager to report the results of the meeting to his department and was disappointed to find it nearly empty. All he found was a message from Roger Brandon's secretary stating that the Johnson kidney damage case had been settled out of court. Since there was no one there in whom he could confide, he went home feeling deflated. At supper, he reported on the meeting to Janet whose reaction was, "Thank God that's over and done. Now we can change the topic of discussion around here."

"I don't appreciate your attitude," Jim replied. "Someone ought to own up to the fact that Amstel was an unsatisfactory candidate because he was a poor excuse for a scientist, not because the Pharmacology department was creating a fuss."

"That's the difference between how things ought to be and how they are," Janet wisely stated. "If you don't recognize that, you're really living in an ivory tower."

"You're probably right, but I still find it distressing that so few seem to see our side. I'm not getting any satisfaction out of this."

"What was your objective?"

Jim hesitated a moment and then said. "To prevent Amstel, with his lousy science and cynical attitudes from leading our department."

"Well, you've done that! To expect a reward for doing that is childish."

Jim recognized that his wife was right. He wanted a pat on the back from some all-powerful parental figure to let him know he had done a fine job and restore the confidence which he had lost during his time on the Search Committee. He needed a diversion, something to combat the thoughts which had traversed, circled, crisscrossed and popped up here and there in his brain during his waking hours. He'd had dreams too of endless meetings. During one stretch he'd met all of one day, dreamed of meetings all night, and continued meeting the next day. Even to the most avid meeting fancier, which he was not, this would have been too much.

Krecke lived in a small apartment two blocks from the hospital. He lived alone by choice, as he was particular about the way in which he kept his things. As a college student, he had lived in a dormitory. He had even had roommates for a period, but such relationships were not to his liking. His standards of proper behavior and neatness were too narrow and he would invariably end up in some disagreeable fuss which he eventually learned to avoid by living alone. He wasn't lonely. There simply wasn't time. He'd so much to learn and do if he were to remain on schedule. He was bound he'd be tops in his profession by the time he was thirty-five. He was now thirty-one and about to be the chief resident on Obstetrics and Gynecology. With the pyramid system, that had taken some doing. In this system, there is a yearly pruning of the house staff as they progress up the ladder from intern to resident and eventually to the peak of the pyramid, the chief resident. You have to be good to get that one, he thought. Good, yes, but so much more. As chief resident you really run the service. Day to day decisions regarding patients, house staff, bed disposition—all these are in the hands of the chief resident especially if the department head trusts you. The next step up from there is usually an invitation to be on the attending staff or even the faculty after you become Board Certified by passing tough specialty examinations.

He had done well so far through hard work, brains and singleness of purpose. Once he had made up his mind, nothing stopped him. If something or someone stood in his way, he would figure a way around the obstacle. When he'd been an assistant resident competing for a residency with a formidable opponent, he'd tipped the scales in his own favor by the simple expedient of getting his opponent drunk early one evening when both drew late duty. It could be argued that one ought not drink when one is going on duty, but there had been a sudden change in scheduling of which the opponent had been unaware. Krecke knew of it and had taken advantage of the change by feeding his opponent bourbon and ginger ale while he drank only ginger ale. Had his victim been canny, she would have wondered why Krecke had invited her for drinks, but she was a recent transfer and had a small crush on her fellow assistant resident whom she had not yet gotten to know. For that matter, there were relatively few who did truly know Daniel Krecke. He was handsome in a dark and brooding way. He was considered extremely competent but definitely a loner. Few had experienced his odd outbursts as had Bill Michaelson or called forth his irrational degree of wrath. Most of the medical faculty considered him somewhat odd in that he'd seldom socialize.

Jake Bourne didn't like Krecke. He found him competent and advanced him because of his present house staff Krecke was the most deserving. Yet Jake did not feel at ease with Krecke. He had partially made up his mind that when the time came he would recommend Krecke highly for an attending faculty position elsewhere. He could do this as the man was technically good. He could not really put his finger on his dissatisfaction with his next chief resident. It was a faint nagging impression, but it would not go away.

Krecke's opinion of his chief, Jake Bourne was neither good nor bad. He recognized his talents as a technician and learned from him. He abhorred Jake's outgoing and raucous nature so contrary to his own. As with most figures of authority whose position was superior to his own, he considered Bourne a stepping-stone toward his own career goals to be used accordingly. He had considered shooting for Jake's job, but the man was too young to await his retirement. Ousting Jake would be extremely difficult, so Krecke, too, was looking outside for advancement. Still, if he played his cards right, no one was invincible. He was thinking thus when he became aware of a knocking at his door. Who would it be knocking at this hour? he wondered. Eight o'clock wasn't that late, but visits to his apartment were rare. Probably some idiot looking for another apartment. He opened the door and was surprised to see a young woman who looked vaguely familiar.

"Dr. Krecke?" she questioned.

"Yes, what at can I do for you?"

"I'd like to talk with you. May I come in?"

Krecke thought, She probably needs an abortion. Why the hell can't these idiots with "crotch fever" protect themselves instead of making extra work and trouble? He motioned to a couch. "Please, sit down."

After they were both seated, he was startled by her question.

"What do you have against Bill Michaelson?"

It took several seconds for him to place the name. When he did, he began to fume. "What business is that of yours? Are you his wife?"

"No, but I'm a friend who works with him in Dr. Kulps laboratory."

Now he remembered. He'd seen her in the hospital cafeteria, one of many technicians who seemed to waste an inordinate amount of time there.

"How does that give you the right to barge in here and ask stupid questions that are not your concern?"

"I wasn't aware of barging anywhere, and injustice is everyone's concern," she calmly answered."

A goddamn do gooder, he thought, and very cool. "I am not aware of any injustice done Mr. Michaelson. Has he been crying on your shoulder?"

"Dr. Krecke, I did not come here to play games with you. Bill is a friend of my husband, Andy Beardsley and I, and from what I can glean, it would appear that you may be treating him unfairly."

Krecke immediately remembered Andy Beardsley. He was the student present the night he'd spared that poor couple the burdens of expensive care of the meningocele. Was he to be blackmailed? If so, he possibly could be vulnerable. He'd better be careful.

"In what way is he treated unfairly? Can you document any of this?"

Donna had not missed the effect Andy's name had on Krecke. He paled visibly and though his arrogant manner had not changed, she was certain she had delivered a strong message. She decided to play a trump. "I don't really suppose a charge of unfairness of a house officer towards a student could be documented easily, but other things might be. Pathology keeps good records."

Kreck's mouth tightly sealed. A tremor was visible in his jaw muscles and his expression was one of fierce concentration. It was like he had gone into a trance. What was in pathology's records? he wondered. He had wanted to know but owing to the press of work, he'd not looked. Besides, looking might have appeared suspicious. Is this girl bluffing? I do not think so, he thought.

"What exactly do you want of me?" he finally asked.

"Only that you leave Michaelson alone and that he gets a passing grade in OB."

"You are trying to blackmail me!"

"Call it what you will, Dr. Krecke, just be sure Michaelson passes." She rose to let him know their visit was at an end.

Krecke continued to bite his lower lip and sat, not seeming to notice Donna had risen. Slowly he looked up at her and seemed to relax.

"Does Mr. Michaelson or your husband know you're here?"

A chill went through Donna. Krecke's sudden change of manner and his question frightened her. Now she paled. Her sudden fear was not lost on Krecke.

When he realized she was suddenly terrified by him, he said with disdain, "For God's sake, Mrs. Beardsley, what sort of monster do you take me for? I won't hurt you. I may be ahead of my time as regards some things best left unsaid, but I value healthy human life. I merely asked whether Michaelson and Andy knew of your visit to determine how safe our secret is. I don't like Michaelson. He's a smart ass but he's one of many. If I could flunk him,I would: but in his case he's too bright, and flunking him would only mean we'd get him back next year." He rose. "Do they know you are here?" he repeated.

Donna was still hesitant. "Perhaps, that is none of your business."

"Suit yourself," Krecke replied with a grin and let her out into the night.

The next day Jim Kulp tried to talk Rodney into playing golf with him. He was unsuccessful and Rodney reminded him that, as Tony was still on vacation, Jim had better attend the remainder of the department heads' meeting.

"Hell, there won't be anything important discussed, just odds and ends."

"You had better attend!" Rodney insisted and his forceful manner made Jim wonder whether Rodney knew something he didn't.

"I guess you are right," he reluctantly admitted.

Before going to the meeting Jim checked his laboratory and was pleased to find things progressing nicely. The experiments with powdered glass had worked and were easily repeated and thus confirmed. Bill Michaelson appeared happier and more relaxed than he had ever seen him. Donna seemed in a very good mood as well, and Jim wondered what was going on to produce so much joy?

In contrast to his own mood of now mild frustration at attaining the right end for the wrong reason, their apparent happiness slightly depressed him. He realized it was envy and he looked forward to an end of academic politics and a return to research. He had planned to take some vacation, but even that didn't cheer him up. He enjoyed going on vacation following work well done, as with his present lab experiments; but not with loose ends still dangling as in the Search Committee's task.

The meeting took place in the same hospital board room. Today Jim was more relaxed. The proceedings were dull and routine and he had a chance to look around and appreciate what an attractive room it was. The walls were elegantly paneled with a light brown to reddish wood. Large chandeliers hung from a clean white ceiling. Several windows looked out on the lush lawn and flower beds which decorated the front of the hospital. The room, light and airy, was in keeping with the tone of today's meeting. Jim's mind drifted though he was able to follow the sense of the discussions enough to realize his full attention was not needed. Time passed quickly and the meeting was drawing to an uneventful close when the Dean asked if there was anything further to be discussed prior to adjournment.

Dr. Dennis Flagler, the newly appointed chief of Pediatrics, waved his hand. He was sitting across the table from Jim, and something familiar caught Jim's attention.

"Mr. Dean," Flagler said as he lifted a notebook off a pile of papers stacked before him. Even upside down Jim recognized them immediately—Amstel's five publications. Jim's heart raced in his chest. Oh God, what now, he thought.

"I have read these papers," Flagler continued, "and I would move to untable yesterday's motion and then move to bring Dr. Amstel here as the Chairman of Pharmacology."

Jim was dumbfounded. When it had been announced that Flagler had accepted the chair in Pediatrics, much was made of his abilities as a researcher. How could he think those papers were acceptable?

"Is there a second to untable Dr. Crane's motion to table discussion of Dr. Amstel?" the Dean asked. Dr. Crane, himself seconded the motion. There was an ample majority to untable the motion in the vote that followed. It was now obvious to Jim that behind the scenes actions were being taken while he assumed the matter was closed.

"Do you now wish to make your motion to bring Dr. Amstel here?" the Dean asked Flagler.

"I do," was the answer, and the motion was made and seconded.

"Is there discussion?" asked the Dean. Several hands shot up including Jim's. The Dean called on Dr. Fraser, chief of Surgery.

Fraser rose and in his usual calm and quiet voice said, "Despite the efforts of this Search Committee, I for one, cannot believe this particular candidate is the only man in this country who would be satisfactory for this position. In point of fact, in view of the feelings of the department he would lead, he is quite unsatisfactory. I think it would be a grave error to try to bring him here under these circumstances." He sat down.

"Dr. Bourne." have you something to say?" the Dean asked.

Jake rose "I heartily agree with Fraser. Let's look some more."

"Jim? Your hand was up. Do you have something to add?" Dean Mackenzie asked.

Jim rose. Things moved so rapidly he'd not had time to become nervous. "Has any of you read these papers?" he asked. He looked around the room trying to catch the eyes of certain department heads. Most would not return his glance. One who did was Al Crane. "Al" Jim queried, "yesterday you tabled discussion on Amstel feeling as Dr. Fraser does. Today you seconded the untabling. Did your reading of the papers lead you to that?"

Crane looked thoughtful. "No, Jim I've not yet read the papers. It's doubtful I ever will, but I'm going to have to vote." Jim sat down shaking his head in confusion.

There was little further discussion. The motion was brought and, much to Jim's surprise and relief, it was soundly defeated. The Dean looked unhappy, but Jim could not tell whether he was more so than usual. The meeting was adjourned.

On his way out Jim stopped to talk with Mary White.

"I thought Dennis Flagler was supposed to be such a hot researcher. How could he think well of those papers, Mary?"

Mary, whom Jim had never heard an improper word pass her lips, replied "That son of a bitch knows those papers are awful. He just owes John Block a favor."

Isn't anyone honest, he wondered? He recalled a time when Bob Mettlar had chided him for stating that honesty was an absolute. Jim had said, "You were either honest or you weren't."

"Nonsense," Bob had replied. "Have you never taken a pencil home from work?" Jim realized that Bob was right and like most things in life there were degrees of honesty.

Whether anyone was honest or not, the Amstel candidacy was probably a dead issue unless the Dean chose to ignore the advice of his department heads.

It was still early and feeling hungry, Jim went to the hospital cafeteria for a snack. He saw Rodney and Linda Koster alone at a table and went to join them, He'd known Linda only slightly but had heard Rodney speak of her in connection with Marie's illness.

"May I join you?" he asked.

"Please do." Linda replied.

"The news is good, Rod, the advisory group rejected Amstel flat out!"

"They damned well should have, but thank God anyway," was his reply. He didn't seem very happy.

"I'd hoped the news would please you," Jim said.

"It does," Rodney replied. "I'm just worn down."

"I have some news," Linda allowed in a teasing way.

"Oh, what's that?' asked Jim.

"I'll be leaving for a new job this fall, and I'm very excited about it. I can't get much of a positive response from our serious friend here, though," she said, nodding toward Rodney.

Rodney grinned, "I just hate to see you go, Linda. Marie has so depended on you."

"I know, Rod, but she's strong; she'll make out and so will you," she added with a knowing look at Rodney. "For some time now, I've begun to realize that I need something less emotionally draining than my job has been. I thought I was tough. Some experiences I've had this past year taught me I'm not tough enough. When this opportunity came along, I grabbed it. I'll be working for a company that's making and selling dialyzers and dialysis equipment. That way I'll use my training, but I'll no longer be personally responsible for patients."

"Will that be enough to keep you happy?" asked Rodney.

"I won't know if I don't try, will I? Besides I can always come back to nursing. Good dialysis nurses are hard to find, and Peter will give me a good recommendation."

They both wished her luck and Rodney could already notice a lessening of tension in Linda which spoke well for her decision. That evening Rodney broke the news to Marie. He also noticed a lessening of tension in her, not in response to his news of Linda of which she was already aware, but he was sensitive to some change in Marie he had not noted till that very evening.

That morning in the clinic Linda had taken Marie aside told her of her decision to leave Wilder. She had also told Marie other things, among them of Rodney's whereabouts the night of the student faculty picnic. She stressed his high alcoholic consumption and that he had passed out. She implied he was too drunk for sex but that he was too embarrassed to talk about the night at her apartment to Marie. She did admonish Marie that if she wanted Rodney to remain faithful, she had best get her sexual act together. If she spared herself a bit more she might have more to give Rodney. The choice was hers. Something in Linda's tone carried a conviction the same speech given by Dr. Markley had not. Marie took it to heart and planned to demand more of Rodney but give more at the same time. It would not be easy, but she would try. Rodney had adjusted to the fact that the Pharmacology Department chairmanship at Wilder was not to be his. Someone high up didn't want him. Hell, there were other schools. He'd keep his options open.

"Will we be able to leave as planned Thursday morning?" Janet Kulp asked Jim that same evening. He planned to attend a conference in New Hampshire the following week and was taking his family along to camp nearby. When the conference was over they would camp and vacation through Canada.

"Things seem to be quieting down. I don't see why we can't get off," he ventured.

Their camping trailer and station wagon was packed the next day, and Jim was able to get most of his work done. His conference talk, on insulin adsorption to various surfaces, required slides for projection; and, though they had been promised earlier, were now to be ready Thursday morning at ten.

"Not a problem," said Jim. "We'll pick them up on our way out of town."

That night Jim was awakened by a nightmare. He dreamt he had been summoned to attend a third meeting of the department heads. The Dean, John Block, and Dennis Flagler were the only others in attendance. The Dean explained that this small group constituted a legitimate quorum whereas the previous meeting, in which Sidney Amstel had been rejected, was improperly conducted. The grounds for this alarming pronouncement were buried deep in a volume of <u>Robert's Rules of Order</u> from which the Dean patiently read long paragraphs to the assembled group. John and Dennis would gravely nod assent as they listened. Jim, who was making a serious attempt to understand was bewildered and terrified. His questions, to gain clarification, were ignored; and, the disdain manifest in the stares he received from the other three participants, silenced his attempts. He awaited the inevitable reconsideration of Amstel with steadily increasing tension till finally he was propelled into wakefulness. He was reassured to find Janet fast asleep beside him, and marveled at his own reactions to the crazy dream: sweating and a rapid heart beat.

Once fully awake, he could not go back to sleep. It was too early to arise and he did not want to disturb Janet, so he lay still considering all that had happened this past academic year. It had been a fascinating and enlightening year. His research had begun to move, his involvement in medical school politics, though frustrating, had been instructive. He'd seen the operations of powerful selfish men blocked by the system. Or were they? He'd learned how little common sense and logic played in the decisions which ran things. That lesson dismayed him, but there it was, like it or not.

He lay for some time sorting and sifting through the events, trying to summarize it all as one did in a scientific publication. You make observations and try to conclude what they mean.

He was suddenly struck by the thought that at this very moment Block or Shane might be going through the exact same exercise. Given the same set of facts he was sure the conclusions drawn would markedly differ. He derived some satisfaction from the idea that they, too, might be having trouble sleeping until he decided that thought was nonsense. Block, Root and Shane seemed to thrive on conflict. What had seemed to take a toll on his departmental associates who were unused to political bickering, appeared to be a way of life for many members of the Search Committee.

What, then is the difference between these people, the watchers and the tellers, those who let things happen and those who try to make things happen?

If you are a seeker of truth, you must be a watcher. Your approach must never inject matter which will alter the truth you are seeking, else you'll be led to some other truth: not the one you are seeking. The history of mankind is filled with examples of barking up the wrong tree. Until some seeker and watcher finds the right tree, the error goes unnoticed and is compounded. In his present state of mind, the most depressing part of it all was that he was beginning to realize the truth of Amstel's assertion that very few give a damn. In that unhappy mood he finally dropped off to sleep.

On Thursday morning, they finished their last minute chores, piled into their station wagon and headed into the medical complex. Jim parked and entered the Pharmacology Department office where the secretary had collected his morning mail including the slides. There were three envelopes which he stuffed into his rear pant's pocket. He opened the box of slides and, using the daylight streaming in the window and a hand viewer, surveyed the eight slides which appeared satisfactory. He said his good-byes and hurried off to the station wagon. He climbed into the driver's seat, and they were off on their vacation.

Driving down the road they were singing, shouting and generally expressing happiness when Jim remembered the letters.

"Jan," he asked, get those letters out of my pocket, please?" He eased his body slightly off the seat to make it easier for her.

She grasped the letters and in the spirit of the moment sang out, "What have we hear? Epistles for the good Doctor James B. Kulp M.D.Ph.D. Pray tell me sir, what should I do with them?"

"Read them to me."

"Oh, Jim, can't they wait?"

"No, honey read them now. It could be something that needs immediate attention."

"That's what worries me. I don't want to think about Wilder for a month."

"Read them Janet," he implored.

"All right, Dr. Kulp." She opened the first letter. "It's from the <u>Journal of Biophysical Phenomena.</u>"

"Never heard of it," Jim admitted.

"Dear sir," she read aloud, "'the <u>Journal of Biophysical Phenomena,</u> is a new journal soon to be published dealing with physical phenomena as they may affect biological systems. The editors of the <u>British Journal of Endocrinology</u> have contacted me concerning certain research work done by you and described in a manuscript submitted to them for publication. I have had the pleasure of reading your manuscript and would be happy to print it as is in my first issue of the journal to be published some time this fall.' The rest is just detail, Jim It's signed by Jerome V. Cooperman."

On hearing that name, Jim let out a long whistle. "He's a Nobel prize winner. That ought to be a good journal."

"The fact that he's bright enough to recognize the worth of your work tells me all I need to know about him," Janet beamed.

"Hey, that'll be a quick publication. In time to include in my grant renewal application. Hot dog! Things are looking up. What other news do you have?"

"This letter seems to be a wedding announcement. 'Mr. and Mrs. Edward C. Marsh request the honor of your presence at the marriage of their daughter, Marian Redford Marsh...'"

"Who the hell's that?"

"Isn't Donna's maiden name Marsh?"

"I think you're right, but I've never even met her sister. Why us? Who is she marrying?"

"William Mitchell Michaelson!"

"No!" Jim shook his head in surprise. "Bill getting married! I wonder how that happened. I've been so busy with the search, I don't know what's going on right under my nose."

"If she's half as nice as Donna, he's a lucky guy."

"He's a good man, Jan. That's great! What's the last letter?"

Janet opened the final envelope. It contained a short letter which she read to herself and giggled. The giggle turned to laughter, but Jim sensed more nervousness than mirth in her laugh.

"What's so funny?" he asked. He repeated the question when his question went unanswered as she continued laughing. She attempted to hand him the letter without a word of explanation.

"For God's sake, you want to get us killed. You know I can't drive and read at the same time." He pulled off the road at the next convenient spot and took the letter. It was addressed to members of the Search Committee. He'd received the last carbon copy as his name was last on the list. The memorandum read:

Memo: To Pharmacology Search Committee Members
From: Francis R. Mackenzie, Dean

The purpose of this memorandum is to inform you officially that the Faculty Advisory Committee by a majority vote did not accept the recommendation of Dr. Sidney B. Amstel for the Chairmanship of the Pharmacology Department.

For many reasons it would seem wise to continue the same committee and I hope that each of you will be willing to serve in this capacity. Dr. Shane will soon be contacting you in regard to a suitable time for a meeting. I have asked that I might meet with you initially for a few minutes because it is essential that certain ground rules be laid down with the full understanding and acceptance by members of the committee.

"Oh no!" His head slumped down on the steering wheel. Janet was still laughing quietly but her laugh could have been mistaken for a sob.

"Are we in New Hampshire, Mommy?" their youngest asked.

"Not yet,dear," Janet answered.

Jim slowly raised his head from the steering wheel. His grim expression was filled with some of his old fire.

"'Non illegitimus carborundum,'" he mumbled.

"What's that supposed to mean?" Janet demanded.

"Don't let the bastards grind you down," he explained, laughing as he drove on to and down the highway.

ABOUT THE AUTHOR

Dr. Hill received his medical and graduate degrees from Columbia University. He spent the major portion of his professional life in medical research and teaching on the faculty of the University of North Carolina Medical School until he joined the Becton, Dickinson Research Center where he headed the Department of Biochemistry and Pharmacology. During his professional life, he authored many scientific publications and received an award for excellence in scientific communication. In retirement, he now authors fiction based, in varying degrees, upon his past experiences. Born and raised in the North, he moved to the South in 1952. Having lived more than half of his life in the South he considers himself a darn Yankee rather than a damn Yankee.